Phyllis, Phallus, Genghis Cohen

& OTHER CREATURES I HAVE KNOWN

Phyllis, Phallus, Genghis Cohen

& OTHER CREATURES I HAVE KNOWN

By Fredric L. Frye, DVM, MSc, FIBiol.
Fellow, Royal Society of Medicine

Illustrated by Robert M. Miller, DVM

KRIEGER PUBLISHING COMPANY
MALABAR, FLORIDA
1995

Original Edition 1984
Reprint Edition 1995 with additional material

Printed and Published by
KRIEGER PUBLISHING COMPANY
KRIEGER DRIVE
MALABAR, FLORIDA 32950

Copyright © 1984 by Fredric L. Frye
Reprinted by arrangement

Library of Congress Cataloging-In-Publication Data

Frye, Fredric L.
   Phyllis, Phallus, Genghis Cohen & other creatures I have known /
by Fredric L. Frye : illustrated by Robert M. Miller.
      p.   cm.
   Originally published: Santa Barbara, CA : American Veterinary
Publications, 1984.
   ISBN 0-89464-932-9 (alk. paper)
   1. Frye, Fredric L.   2. Veterinarians—California—Berkeley—
Biography.   I. Title.   II. Title: Phyllis, Phallus, Genghis Cohen,
and other creatures I have known.
SF613.F78A3   1995
636.089′092—dc20
[B]
                                                                94-43399
                                                                CIP
10 9 8 7 6 5 4 3 2

Dedication

To my wife Brucye, and our children Lorraine and Erik, who shared the excitement during my years in clinical practice; to my grandsons Noah and Ian, who are already proving the heritability of their grandfather's curiosity and fondness for animals; and to the memory of my parents Ben and Ann, who displayed great forebearance towards my early interest in animals in general and in reptiles and invertebrates specifically—I *know* that there were times when I gave them reasons to question their decision to have children (at least a son who was inseparable from his menagerie).

Acknowledgments

I never could have written this book without the confidence of my clients who shared their lives with me or without the support of my colleagues and lay staff of the Berkeley Dog & Cat Hospital.

My thanks to Winnifred Madison for her assistance with my original manuscript, and to Roxanne Lapidus who edited the first edition of this book. Eleven years later, with the urging of colleagues to reprint, Robert E. Krieger of Krieger Publishing Company (who has published five of my other books) again showed his confidence in my written words. My gratitude to Elaine Harland, also of Krieger Publishing, who was an ardent supporter of this new reissued edition.

Special appreciation to my wife Brucye, who not only lived through many of these experiences with me, but helped me with every stage of the manuscript. As always, her judgement was solid and her efforts enthusiastically given.

Particular thanks to my colleague, Dr. Robert M. Miller, for his lively cartoons. As fellow veterinarians, we speak the same language!

Table of Contents

All photographic images (except the cover illustration) were made by Fredric L. Frye.

The names of all clients have been changed.

1 | A Herpetologist is Not Someone with Herpes

The telephone rang shrilly in the darkness. Eyes closed, I reached for the instrument.

"This is Dr. Frye," I managed to enunciate.

"Dr. Frye? This is William DeWitt. Sorry to call you so late, but I just got home from a long weekend. It's about my vine snake. I looked in his cage, and he's lying out straight on his back, all stiff."

"Sounds like he's dead."

"But how can I be sure?"

I opened one eye and looked at the clock. It was 1:45 a.m. "Get a long stick and poke him. If he moves, he's alive. If not, he's dead."

"But what if he's dead?"

"You can use him for a walking stick or a chalkboard pointer," I said wearily, and hung up.

The next morning he called back.

"Oh Dr. Frye — about my snake — I thought you'd like to know. When I opened his cage, I could smell a bad smell. He was dead all right."

'Twas a pity he did not use his olfactory sense before making the first call. But I suppose I should be grateful he did not call me back again that night with his findings!

Night calls were an accepted plague in our veterinary practice. But the most bizarre ones always seemed to concern reptiles and their owners. Do reptiles confer on their keepers a propensity towards strange behavior, or are people who like reptiles simply eccentric?

9

Since I am a confessed reptile fancier, I have never examined this question too closely.

One of my herpetological clients was Howard. He wore thick glasses that enabled him to distinguish images; he was legally blind. He had been a physicist at the University of California here in Berkeley, and his conversation had a way of always digressing into theoretical physics — charged particles, ergs, masses accelerating at something "per second per second." Perhaps this is why he was so vague about real time — our prosaic twenty-four hours, with clocks and schedules and appropriate hours for doing things.

One night I received an agitated call from Howard. "Dr. Frye, this is Howard Martin. I was just out in the hills, searching for specimens, and I've been bitten. I'm quite sure it was a rattlesnake."

"How long ago did this happen?"

"About an hour ago. I came straight home, but it took me awhile to find my way."

"Well, call a taxi, man, and get to the emergency room. Or call an ambulance."

"I can't do that. I don't want to go to the emergency room."

"What? Why not?"

"They'll ask me how it happened, you know."

"Well?"

"If I tell them I was groping around in the dark under stones, out there in the hills, they might try to have me put away." Coming from Howard, this was a rare flash of insight.

"You have to get medical help. This is serious."

"Couldn't you treat me? I'd prefer it."

"Absolutely not. I'm not licensed to treat humans. You've got to get to the emergency room, and fast."

"Well, could you call them up first, and tell them what to do?"

"Okay, okay. I'll call. Now you get on over there — fast!"

No veterinarian in his right mind would call a physician and "tell him what to do," but I did call the emergency room and explain the situation.

The physician on duty had never treated a case of snakebite, so my call was fortuitous. Since I was the consultant on reptiles to the Steinhart Aquarium in San Francisco's Golden Gate Park, I was familiar with their protocol for treating venomous snakebites. This included calling Dr. Findlay E. Russell, an international expert on reptile envenomation, who lived in Arizona.

I called the aquarium's night-duty engineer, who gave me Dr. Russell's number. I reached Dr. Russell, who then called the emergency room in Berkeley, and spoke directly with the physician attending Howard.

Howard made an uneventful recovery, and came under the care of a psychiatrist. His interest in reptiles was unabated, however.

A few years after his brush with mortality, Howard called me on a Sunday evening.

"Dr. Frye, this is Howard Martin. I have an emergency with one of my pythons. Can I bring him in now?"

"What kind of an emergency?"

"I'll tell you when I see you. Can you see us now? I'll call a taxi."

I arrived at the hospital before Howard did and pulled the charts on his various reptiles since I wasn't sure which one he was bringing. Outside, I heard the squeal of brakes, and looking out the window, I saw a taxi at the curb.

I unlocked the front door and went out to meet Howard. The taxi driver sat limply behind the wheel, not moving. Slowly the rear door opened, and Howard emerged holding a blood-soaked handkerchief to the lower part of his face. Blood was streaming down his chin and onto his shirt front. As soon as he stepped free of the cab, the driver shot off, not waiting for his fare.

I ushered Howard inside. In his hand was an overnight suitcase. "Tell me what has happened!"

"Well, I was looking for my new African rock python. I knew he was in the apartment, but I couldn't find him. So I was feeling my way around when WHAM! — he hit me right here."

His nine-foot "pet" — a species that is known for its aggressiveness — had landed a well-aimed strike on the lower part of Howard's face. (How many feet does a striking python travel "per second per second," I wonder? Surely something comparable to a charged particle!) The well-developed, recurved teeth had laid open Howard's lower lip.

Leaving the snake in the overnight suitcase where Howard had stuffed it, we drove to the emergency room, where nine stitches were placed in the hapless victim's lip.

Two weeks later, a similar scenario was enacted, this time involving Howard's *upper* lip.

I had all but forgotten about Howard when, about a year later, I saw his name in my appointment book. In the past, he had often made appointments that he forgot to keep, but this time he showed.

He seemed dejected as he looked myopically through his thick glasses.

"Dr. Frye, I've tried and tried with Petruchio." (The infamous python.) "I just don't understand it."

"What's he done now?"

"Well, you know I have a cat." He gulped. "Had a cat. A nice soft cat named Imogene."

"Yes?"

"Well, I have reason to believe — that is, now I'm *sure* — Petruchio — he *ate* Imogene!" Howard blinked rapidly.

"He ate---? Ah! I see. Well — uh — that *is* very distressing." Words seemed to elude me.

"So I was wondering — do you think you could find a good home for Petruchio? A zoo, maybe, where he would be safe?"

I agreed heartily, and we shook hands. That was the last time I saw Howard.

My "fame" as a herpetological veterinarian was sometimes less than gratifying. One night the emergency phone rang its way into my slumbers at 3 a.m.

"Hello, Doc Frye? This is Eddie Cahill, disc jockey here at KJAZ. Listen, we had a call an hour ago about a sick iguana. The guy wanted us to ask the listeners where he could get help for his pet iguana. Somebody called in with your name."

He waited expectantly, sure of being thanked for being the bearer of this good news. It is fortunate that my immediate reply about a sick iguana at 3 a.m. was not broadcast over the air. I was still groggy — I had already had several bona-fide emergencies that night.

A moment later the lizard's owner was on the line. No, he could not wait till 8 a.m. (a scant five hours away); the creature had already been sick for three weeks. Resigning myself to my fate, I agreed to meet the fellow at 4 a.m. sharp, figuring it would take him an hour to drive over from San Francisco.

I dressed and drove the three miles from our home in Kensington to Berkeley, arriving at ten of four. I slumped down in the receptionist's chair and waited. Four o'clock came and went. All was quiet in the wards. I slumped lower, opening an eye occasionally as a car went by or to check the clock on the wall. Four-thirty.

I cursed all iguanas and their owners, the radio station, and the sadist who had joyfully called in my name. Whatever it was could have waited till 8 a.m. Would a person call out their physician or dentist at such an hour? Would they call their friendly plumber in the middle of the night? Not a chance! *The plumber charges more for his time!*

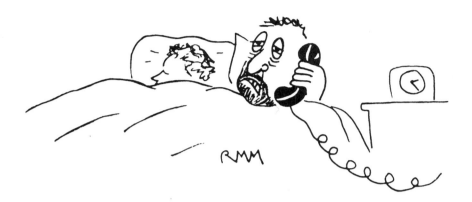

At 5:15 I locked the door behind me and navigated home. I hoped to catch two or three hours of sleep before returning to work. I tried to remember if any delicate surgery were scheduled for that day. If only it were on the owner of the iguana!

Veterinary emergency clinics are now a reality in many communities, and have greatly improved the practice conditions of veterinary medicine. No more slumbers interrupted by the heart-stopping shrill of the telephone. No more fumbling with buttons and shoe laces in the dark. No more dangerous drives in a semi-conscious state. No more false alarms. Just a friendly answering service voice that says "The hospital is closed. Please call the veterinary emergency clinic at the following number. They are open from 6 p.m. to 8 a.m. You can reach the doctor at the office in the morning."

On the other hand, my notoriety as an expert in treating reptiles sometimes brought a touch of excitement and even glamor to our veterinary hospital. One such episode involved a large indigo snake with an unusual name.

In the 1960's, "topless" dancing had become a big attraction in the tourist joints of San Francisco's North Beach area. (San Francisco's Twin Peaks are a bona-fide landmark, but during that era they were rivaled by a second set of "twin peaks" — those boasted by Carol Doda, a lass of siliconized megawomanhood, and the reigning topless dancer!)

One evening I received an emergency call. "Hello, Dr. Frye, this is Barry Steinberg. I'm the agent for Tara, the dancer who's featured at "The Spotlight" in North Beach. You may have heard of her act?"

"No, I can't say that I have."

"Well, it's real classy. Not just another topless number. She has this snake, see? A big black one. And she comes out, and I mean she's a real looker, and knows how to play it to the audience. So she's got this snake all coiled around her. She calls him 'Playtex.' You know — 'Playtex, the living bra.' That's the name of the act — 'The Incredible Tara and Playtex the Living Bra.'" He paused for breath, and I listened, spellbound.

"So anyway, he twines all around her, and she — I mean she really socks it to the audience. They go wild. But the trouble is, she's been noticing that Playtex isn't feelin' so good lately. Not too lively. Just sorta hangs there. So you gotta fix him up, Doc. She can bring him over right away. But he's gotta be in the act tonight. Without him, it's nothin'."

Understandably, I could hardly wait to make the acquaintance of Playtex and Tara. I examined the former, and had to be content with just looking at the latter. She was, indeed, a remarkable specimen of womanhood. As for poor Playtex, he had a severe case of ulcerative stomatitis, a serious disease of snakes.

"I'm afraid you'll have to leave him here for a few days," I said, looking down into her heavily fringed eyes.

"Are you sure, doctor? I really need him. Without him, my act is pretty flat."

I could hardly believe that, but as a professional, I decided I must stick with scientific, medical arguments. I finally convinced her to leave the snake with us.

Somehow, word of Playtex's hospitalization reached Herb Caen, whose daily column in the San Francisco Chronicle was an institution. By the next day, all of San Francisco knew of it, and our phone began to ring off the hook. That afternoon a florist's truck pulled up outside, and a spray of pink carnations in a milk-white vase was delivered for Playtex, from the proprietor of "The Spotlight."

Playtex responded rapidly to treatment, and was discharged after a few days, again attended by much publicity. I had the feeling that Tara's agent had been just as busy as I had, rendering emergency service to the situation!

Not all of my cases were so spectacular. In fact, one of the very first cases I treated in private practice was a common garden snail. Though not a reptile, and hardly exotic, it was brought to me.

"This is my pet snail, Cleo," said the child, holding out a jar. "His shell got cracked when I dropped him on the sidewalk. But the rest of him is fine. Can you fix him?"

Her mother interrupted. "I hope you don't find this too ridiculous, Dr. Frye. We've tried to give her other snails, but she's particularly attached to this one. Is there anything to be done?"

I looked down into the intent young face. "Well, Andrea, Cleo has had quite a bad accident, but I *might* be able to fix him. You leave him with me for a few days, and I'll see what I can do."

Later that day, I removed the snail from the jar and looked at it. It looked like any other snail, and it would have been easy to replace it with one of the many in my own garden. But somehow, I could not do that.

I gently elevated the depressed fragments of the shell, and removed the loose debris from the wounds. Then, using epoxy resin glue, I cemented the fragments back in their original shape. This task took about thirty minutes, and when finished, the shell looked almost normal, except for being shiny where it was mended. I kept the snail in a jar in my office for a day or two, to make sure it would survive the operation.

It was with great pleasure that I called my young client and told her that Cleo was ready to go home. The snail lived a hearty six months more after its shell repair. After it died, Andrea kept its empty shell. She put it in a box with cotton, and would often take it out and look at it.

I know this, because Andrea became a staunch client of the Berkeley Dog & Cat Hospital, with a series of other pets as she grew up. She went on to graduate from veterinary school at the University of California at Davis. She has told me that her decision to become a veterinarian was based on her early experiences as my client, starting with Cleo, the snail with the rebuilt shell.

Our practice counted among its patients snakes, lizards, turtles, frogs, toads, alligators, crocodiles, a South American manatee (at Steinhart Aquarium), birds of prey, spiders and scorpions, wolves, foxes and coyotes, a few bears, anteaters, armadillos, llamas, a tapir, and several exotic big cats. With such a patient roster, the potential for severe injuries or zoonotic infections (diseases transmitted from animals to man) was ever present. In the ten years that I was engaged in this practice, I was not injured (except for a rare dog bite or cat scratch), nor was I served with a lawsuit, although the ingredients for several abounded. However, a few "close calls" would occasionally remind me that vigilance was essential.

One Saturday morning, a young couple with an adult Indian cobra came into the hospital, seeking care for the snake's respiratory infection. The cobra was confined in a flimsy pillowcase.

It seems unbelievable that they were not aware of the danger to which they were exposing themselves, and me. The standard method for carrying poisonous snakes is in a reinforced canvas bag, inside a wooden box.

They deposited the pillowcase on the exam table, and I began to ask them the snake's health history. We were discussing its diet when the girl leaned on the exam table and put her hand down on the pillowcase.

The enormous, explosive HISSS! that filled that small room is something I shall not soon forget. I had heard that sound outdoors in Thailand and Pakistan, and in the noisy environments of zoos and aquaria, but never in such close quarters. It was like the sound of steam escaping from a huge locomotive.

"Be careful!" I barked, pushing her away from the table.

She looked at me and shrugged. "I don't think he'd bite me," she said. "Not through the pillowcase."

When the cobra and its owners had left, I ruminated for awhile on Darwin's theory of natural selection. In nature, the truly stupid or incompetent individuals are winnowed out of the gene pool — they can't compete, and die off before reproducing their defects. In *Homo sapiens* (so called), survival of the fittest no longer operates with such certainty. It is a frightening prospect on which to ponder.

I was passing through the outer office as Hattie, our receptionist, talked on the phone. "I see, Mr. Brown. Well, what kind of a snake is it?" There was a long pause, and Hattie grimaced at me.

"You'd rather not say? Well, can you give me an idea of how big it is?" Another pause. "No? Well, can you at least tell me what the complaint is? No? Well, just a moment, I'll see if Dr. Frye will see you."

This conversation was not unusual. *Nominally,* it is against the law for unlicensed people to keep venomous snakes and lizards in California. (The state Fish and Game Department issues permits to zoos and bona-fide research centers; a private person applying for such a permit would simply be inviting confiscation of the creature.) In our practice, when a person refused to give information on the phone, it was usually out of fear of being reported for illegal possession of a dangerous or endangered species.

I had fought my own inner moral battle about this situation, and had concluded that my first duty was to the creature, which meant not scaring off its owner. We saw a number of contraband creatures: cobras, kraits, coral snakes, gila monsters, rattlesnakes and boom-slangs.

I agreed to see young Mr. Brown and his unidentified snake that afternoon at four o'clock.

I entered the exam room at 4 p.m., and froze in my tracks. Coiled on the floor in the center of the room was a nearly six-foot Russell's viper. These serpents are characterized by their long fangs and particularly virulent venom. A well-placed bite from one of these would be almost certainly fatal. The nearest specific antivenin, I knew, was at Steinhart Aquarium, across the bay in San Francisco.

I looked from the coiled serpent to its hirsute young owner. "I'm sorry," I said somewhat breathlessly, "but I won't examine your snake until it is properly restrained. You can use my pole-mounted snake hook there in the corner. Call me when you are ready." I backed out of the room, closing the door behind me.

In a few moments, he called to me. "It's okay, Doc. Everything's cool — you can come in."

I opened the door cautiously and peered in. The young man had one hand firmly around the animal's neck, just behind the lance-shaped head, and the other hand midway down the snake's body.

I entered and hurriedly made my examination and diagnosis. All the while I was mentally calculating how long it would take someone to drive from Steinhart Aquarium to the Berkeley Dog & Cat Hospital — at least forty minutes, under the very best of conditions. Not fast enough.

After that experience, I told Hattie to accept no more venomous animals unless adequate and truthful data were given when the appointment was made, and unless they were brought to the hospital in a safe container.

A third "close call" involved a snake and another of our patients. We had hospitalized an eight-foot Burmese python. Although an adult Burmese python's length and girth make it appear highly dangerous, in general this species is non-aggressive towards humans. This particular snake was an unusually docile and well-fed beast.

Several times daily the creature was removed from his cardboard box for treatment. When he was replaced, we always sealed the box with strapping tape, and placed it inside a stainless steel cage for good measure.

One morning I was making my rounds of that ward with Cheryl, one of our aides. The python's box was in the middle of a bank of cages occupied by various warm-blooded patients. Usually, the snake's distinctive skin pattern was visible through the airholes punched in the carton. Now only an empty darkness was visible.

"Cheryl, where's the python?" I said without much alarm (yet). "I know I put it in the box last evening, and put the box in the cage."

The strapping tape appeared intact, and the air holes seemed too small for a heavy-bodied, eight-foot snake to have squeezed through. Cheryl opened the cage and wordlessly lifted the carton. Empty.

I made a hurried inspection of the lower bank of cages, where two dogs, a cat and a parakeet in its wire cage were separately confined.

"This is something Harry Houdini would've appreciated," I quipped, feeling the first pangs of panic. "All that's missing is the pair of handcuffs."

As I surveyed the uppermost tier of cages, I noticed that the occupant of one, an Abyssinian cat, seemed especially close to the grillwork. In fact, she was pushed right up against it; tufts of her gray fur protruded through.

I opened the door. "Come on, Sheba," I said softly. As I lifted her out, I saw several colored coils of a very contented python, lying peacefully in the back of the cage.

We never did discover how the snake escaped from its box, but apparently, after exploring a bit, it had sought a warm place in which to curl up. Happily, it had not been hungry, for it could easily have killed and devoured the cat. Neither creature was injured, but I can imagine that poor Sheba had had a sleepless night of it!

After that, we insisted that every snake admitted for hospitalization be confined in a lockable terrarium, or be placed in a canvas sack inside a cage. No more Harry Houdini acts, thanks.

Anthony and Bruce were two young herpetologists on my client roster. Their mother did not share their love of amphibians and reptiles, but she was a good sport about their hobby, much as my own mother had been about mine. Gloria would drive her sons on field trips to likely "herping" grounds, and to the Berkeley Dog & Cat Hospital for consultations or help on school science projects.

One day the boys called me. "Hi Dr. Frye — this is Anthony. Guess what Bruce and I just got? A pair of Israeli agama lizards! We traded them from a guy in Chicago! Anyway, they just got here on the United Parcel truck, and we wondered if you could check them out. Before we put them with the rest of the collection, I mean. Mom says she can drive us over anytime this afternoon."

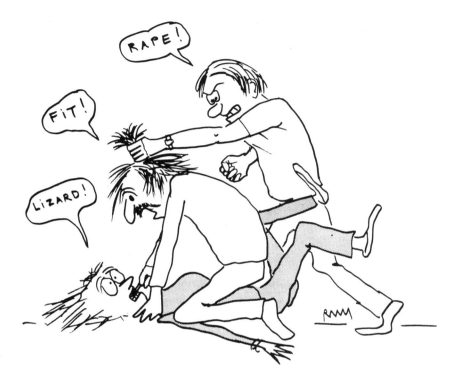

We made a date for 4:30. The appointed time came and went with no sign of the boys, their mother, or the lizards. Some time later, Mike Connelly appeared in the waiting room, beaming broadly. Mike was a client of ours, and a policeman. Hattie ushered him into the back.

"I have a message for you from two young friends of yours," he said cheerfully. "I told them I'd tell you why they missed their appointment."

It seems that on the way to the hospital, the lizards escaped from their box. One of them ran beneath the front seat, and leaped up on Gloria's foot, which was poised invitingly on the accelerator pedal. From this perch, the lizard took refuge inside the woman's trouser leg, and began ascending.

Gloria halted her car in the middle of the street and leaped out, stomping and dancing, trying to dislodge the lizard from the bare skin of her inner thigh. Then, in desperation, she dropped to the pavement and began rolling over and over.

The stopped car in the middle of the street and the writhing woman soon drew a crowd of onlookers. A well-meaning bystander, assuming he was witnessing a seizure, rushed forward to render first aid. To keep the victim from choking on her tongue, he tried to pry her mouth open with a ballpoint pen.

A second Good Samaritan mistook this act for an assault, and leaped into the fray, pummelling the first man with his fists. The onlookers set up a cry for the police.

When the police arrived, the distraught woman was helped to her car, in which privacy she was able to remove her slacks and the lizard. The terrified creature was still alive, although it had lost part of its tail.

No charges were leveled against Gloria for obstructing traffic, nor against the first man for smearing ink on her front teeth, nor at the second man for punching him.

"What on earth were Tony and Bruce doing all this time?" I managed to gasp, between paroxysms of laughter.

"In the car trying to catch the other lizard," grinned Mike. "They were all for continuing on over here, but their mother said she'd had enough for one day." He smiled fondly at the memory of that scene. "I think maybe she was right."

Just another typical day in Berkeley!

2 | Welcome to Berkeley Dog & Cat Hospital

Berkeley is a university town. The University of California campus is at the center of the town, backing up against hillside wilderness, and commanding a view down University Avenue towards the bay, San Francisco, and the Golden Gate.

As a university town, it has long been known for the liberal views and diversity of its population. Among our clients at the Berkeley Dog & Cat Hospital were professors, Nobel laureates, impoverished students, and a generous sprinkling of people whose behavior was beyond the bell-shaped curve of what is considered "normal."

Berkeley Dog & Cat Hospital faces onto Haste Street, a busy thoroughfare of Berkeley. The hospital had been christened in 1907, when the average pet was a dog or cat. Even earlier, this had been the site first of a livery stable, then of a poultry butcher, and later of a large animal hospital serving dairy cattle and horses, including those owned by the police and fire departments in the Oakland and Berkeley area.

The building had survived the 1906 earthquake that had leveled much of San Francisco, and had been remodeled several times since then. My partner, Jean-Paul Cucuel, and I bought the building and the practice in 1966. Three years later, we made extensive renovations, replacing nearly all of the building with a modern hospital facility. We kept the name "Dog & Cat Hospital," though it hardly described the variety of creatures that crossed our threshold!

21

One of my more unusual patients was a furry creature named Anastasia...

As the young, casually attired couple entered the sunlit reception room, they hesitated. The girl was holding a pink cardboard cake box, in which a few small holes had been punched. It dangled from her hand by a string.

"Where should we sit?" her companion said.

To their left was an area enclosed by a railing and gates; it already held two rambunctious terriers and their owner. To their right was a large former aviary, now housing some green iguanas and plants. Next to it was a bench already occupied by a woman with a cat carrier. Loud mewing emanated from the carrier, and now and then a dark paw poked out through a hole.

"Anastasia is in a box, so I guess we should sit where the cat is," the girl said. She turned to the receptionist.

"Do you think Dr. Frye will know what Anastasia's problem is?" she asked in a quavering voice. "She doesn't look quite right to me."

When I entered the examination room I found the tearful girl and her companion, who was now holding the pink box. He handed it to me and put an arm around the girl's shoulders.

I placed the carton on the stainless steel examination table, removed the string, and opened the lid. The bottom of the box was littered with assorted hairy legs, pieces of hairy skin and other body parts — the dismembered remains of what a few hours before had been a vigorous, furry tarantula! Indeed, Anastasia did *not* look quite right!

The owners had noticed that the spider was shedding its skin, which it does at irregular intervals. During a natural molt, the old epidermis splits along its edges as the spider flexes its body, and the creature emerges from its old coat by crawling free. Each leg is, in turn, pulled free of its sleeve of old cuticle. Missing legs, old worn fangs and even the corneas covering the eight eyes are replaced at this time. Quite innocently, the young couple had tried to help their pet, and had tugged at the adherent skin. Unfortunately, in doing so, they had pulled the spider apart.

After I had explained the natural history of spiders in general and tarantulas in particular, the youngsters left to buy another. They phoned later to tell me their new pet was named "Rasputin." They seemed to be well acquainted with pre-Bolshevik Russian history!

That afternoon at Berkeley Dog & Cat Hospital promised to be anything but dull.

My next client was an unscheduled one — a rather derelict young man and his large dog, Sam. Hattie, our jewel of a receptionist, assured me that although I usually referred dermatology cases to one of my junior colleagues, this was one for me to see! The conversation in the reception room had gone something like this:

"Now, what is Sam's problem?"

"Oh, m'dawg has bugs."

"Probably fleas," said Hattie knowingly.

"Naw, fleas jump, and the bugs this critter has, they just kinda *crawl*. Besides, I got 'em too."

During this exchange, he had been alternately digging into his armpits and scratching his crotch.

As I talked to Sam's hirsute and unkempt owner, it emerged that he and the dog shared the same bed. They also shared the same parasite: the human pubic crab louse, *Phthirus pubis,* which is usually

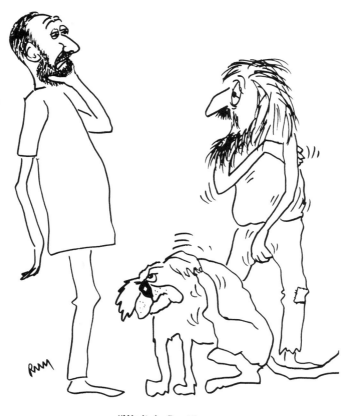

"We itch, Doc!"

confined to human hosts. This case marked the first time since 1919 that an authenticated case of phthiriasis was diagnosed and reported in the veterinary literature.

I dispensed an insecticidal shampoo (to be used by *both* of them), and discussed measures to rid their sleeping quarters of the parasite. When I was through, my client, now scratching more vigorously than ever, offered to shake my hand. Diplomatically, I was in the process of washing with soap and hot water! Nonetheless, for the balance of the afternoon, I, too, was scratching, even though none of the crawlies had actually transferred their allegiance to me!

My next client was a large woman in her early thirties, carrying a moving pillowcase. The history card said she wished a consultation about her boa constrictor's nose.

A cloud of perfume accompanied her into the room, and she deposited the creature on the exam table with much jingling of bracelets.

"This is Bonaparte," she said huskily. "You see here where his nose is all scarred?" She pointed with a red lacquered fingernail. "He was bitten by a rat I fed him a few weeks ago. Now the scar tissue is blocking his nostrils, and he can only breathe through his mouth." She sank gracefully into a chair.

The snake's condition could be repaired by a rhinoplasty, to create two new orifices. I described the procedure, which entails inserting plastic tubing in the new passages so they will not become obliterated by scar tissue as they heal. These are removed after a few weeks.

"That sounds good," the woman said, crossing and recrossing her legs. "I'd like to watch you do it, if possible. I'm a veterinarian too."

"Oh?" I said, surprised. "Which school did you graduate from?"

"Arizona."

"Tuscon or Tempe?"

"Tempe," she said, twirling her bracelets. "But I'm prevented from practicing in California by the State Board of Examiners. Because of my change of status."

By now I was more than a little curious. There are no schools of veterinary medicine in Arizona, and the California Board of Veterinary Medical Examiners needs adequate cause to prohibit someone from practicing. The alleged cause was soon forthcoming.

"It's because of my change of status," she repeated. "I've only recently become a woman."

As she continued her tale, I noted that her hands, feet and features were definitely more masculine than feminine. Moreover, her mannerisms were exaggerated, sometimes to the point of absurdity.

She had undergone transsexual surgery about a year before, and was still receiving hormone therapy.

"Well, about Bonaparte's surgery," I said prosaically when her recital was over, "I don't know exactly when I'll be doing it, so I'm afraid it will be impossible for you to watch." She nodded, twirling her bracelets again. "But I will go over the exact procedure with you when you come in to collect him. And of course you'll receive the professional courtesy discount that we give to all our veterinary colleagues."

She shook my hand. "Thank you, Doctor, I appreciate it." She left gracefully, in a cloud of perfume.

At the reception desk, I heard her asking Hattie for directions to the restroom. On leaving, she stopped again to talk to Hattie.

"Oh these cramps!" the husky voice said. "What a curse we women bear!"

"I know how it is," said Hattie cheerfully.

I had occasion to see Bonaparte's owner several times for postsurgical care of the boa's nose, but I never indicated that I considered her anything but a lady!

The atmosphere at Berkeley Dog & Cat Hospital was fun-loving and "hang-loose." We practiced top-quality medicine and surgery, and I was engaged in various scientific research projects, but none of this interfered with our enjoyment of practical (so-called!) jokes. Whenever we received a new resident veterinarian into our fold, the staff could not resist initiating him with some prank.

One conscientious and well-trained clinician who applied for an opening in our hospital was Dr. Clarke Atwater. From our interviews, we gathered that he also had that other prerequisite for joining our ranks: a good sense of humor. He was hired.

On Clarke's first day with us, I brought my lunch in a paper bag. While he was busy with a patient, I summoned the operating room staff into surgery. We removed my "lunch" from the bag — a rubber plucked chicken, complete with wattles and curled feet. Laying this patient on the operating table, we hooked it up to the automatic positive-pressure respirator so that it was "breathing" rhythmically. A catheter connected to a drip bottle of IV solution was attached to the fowl. Elated with the effect, we draped the patient with the standard green surgical drapes so that only a small section of latex skin was showing.

We gathered gleefully in an adjoining room, and Cheryl knocked excitedly on the door of Clarke's exam room.

"Dr. Atwater! There's a code blue in the surgery prep room!"

Clarke entered the room on the run, jamming his stethoscope into his ears. He bent over the draped form and began moving the stethoscope over it. After a few seconds he paused, straightened, and touched the exposed "skin." Glancing up at us hovering in the doorway, he whipped back the drapes and exposed the disreputable bird.

Clarke joined us in the general laughter. In the ensuing days, he repaid our efforts with generous dividends!

Another young veterinarian, Dr. Dennis Hoeft, joined us after completing a residency at the Animal Medical Center in New York City. In our practice, one of his first patients was a cat with a chronic, incurable disease. The cat declined steadily over several months, although Denny did everything possible for it.

"The poor creature is suffering so," he said to me in exasperation, "but the owner won't let me put it to sleep. We have to wait and watch it die by inches." The situation was obviously painful to him.

The cat finally died in its sleep, to the great relief of all of us on the staff. Denny obtained permission to perform a postmortem examination.

A few weeks earlier, I had happened to turn on the radio to a High Requiem Mass recited by Pope Paul VI. Sensing possibilities, I had quickly switched on my tape recorder.

The day after the cat's demise, Denny lay the wasted cadaver on the postmortem exam table, and prepared to make his investigations. The small room was quiet, except for the clink of instruments. Slipping in unobtrusively, I switched on my tape.

"*Domine Jesu Christe, Rex gloriae, libera animas omnium fidelium defunctorum de poenis inferni et de profundo lacu...*"

His Holiness's sonorous voice reverberated off the walls, filling the small room. Denny, a devout man, sat frozen in mid-knife stroke.

"*Agnus Dei, qui tollis peccata mundi: dona eis requiem sepiternam.*"

Fortunately, Denny, too, had a good sense of humor, and saw my irreverent "ceremonies" as a fitting end to his vain efforts to save the hopeless cat. Everyone on the staff joined in the laughter and the sense of relief.

We veterinarians took turns being "on call" in the evenings, which resulted in many interrupted dinners and rude awakenings. At staff meeting one morning, Clarke Atwater, looking somewhat bleary-eyed, smiled grimly at Jean-Paul and me.

"You won't believe the calls I had last night! You know Nancy Moffat, and her dog Prissy?"

Jean-Paul and I groaned. Nancy Moffat was well known to nearly every veterinarian in the Bay Area. She would go to one for a few times, and then throw a tirade in the waiting room, and threaten to sue. She had exhausted all the practices in San Francisco, and now was favoring us with her custom. She was unstable and had a drinking problem. So far, we had managed to handle her diplomatically but firmly, and there had been no embarrassing scenes in *our* waiting room.

"Okay," said Clarke, "so she's been giving Prissy her heart medicine now for three months. Twice a day, just pop the pill in, no problem.

"So, last night, I'm just sitting down to dinner, and the phone rings. It's Nancy, and she's been drinking. She says she needs advice on how to get the pill down, but then she starts telling me about how bad her landlord is, and how the government is corrupt, and all kinds of other good stuff. Meanwhile, my dinner is getting cold. I tell her again and again how to do it — 'hold the muzzle, put it far back on the tongue, down it goes' — and finally I get rid of her. I start reheating my dinner.

"I'll spare you all the details, but after the third call I begin to keep a *count* of how many times she's calling me. And each time, it sounds like she's had another drink before dialing.

"Okay, are you ready for this? This is call number *nine* in the space of three hours. It's now ten o'clock, and I'm still trying to finish my dinner. I've stopped trying to heat it up; the peas are like pebbles.

"So the phone rings, and she says, 'Dr. Atwater, I shtill can't get Prishy's pill down.'

"By now, I've had it. I say, 'Okay, here's what you can do with that pill. You can take it and shove it up Prissy's —.' And I hang up."

Jean-Paul and I listened, agog. *Here we go,* I thought, *she'll be in the waiting room as soon as the hangover wears off.*

"But that's not all," said Clarke, with great satisfaction. "Here comes the best part! Ten minutes later, I can't believe it, but the phone is ringing again. It's Nancy.

"'Doctor,' she says, 'I *know* what you want me to do. But that damned pill, it keepsh falling out. Beshides, it'sh ruining my m-manicure. Can't I jusht give it the old way?'"

Clarke grinned broadly as we collapsed in helpless mirth. "Let her sue," I gasped between paroxysms. "It was worth it!"

A few days later, I saw Nancy Moffat's name on my list of appointments, and felt some pangs of dread. But her only reference to the incident was to say that she would prefer *not* to have Prissy cared for by our young colleague. Not because of his lack of skill, she admitted, but because she was too embarrassed to face him. Clarke was happy to comply.

Another client who had to be handled delicately by the staff was an obviously disturbed woman who possessed at least two distinct personalities.

One persona was that of an extremely prim lady dressed in high-necked dresses that came below the knees. As such, she referred to her bitch's external genitalia as a "hoo-hoo." Whenever the animal was brought in for an inflammation of this area, we had to refer to it as "hoo-hooitis."

Her second personality was the exact opposite. At these times, she dressed like a low-priced streetwalker, and laced her conversations with four-letter words. Her bitch's "hoo-hoo" was now referred to by a slang synonym for its human counterpart.

Where we had to be on our toes was when, in an animated conversation, the woman would switch back and forth between the two personalities. Her pupils would dilate, and she would become someone else within a moment or two. If one of us missed the transition and used the wrong vocabulary, as sometimes happened, she would turn on us in great offense.

"Doctor, if you must discuss such subjects with me, kindly refer to it as a 'hoo-hoo.' Scientific names embarass me."

"Well, it looks like Mitzi has hoo-hooitis again."

"What? Let's not beat around the bush, damn it! So she's got this crappy stuff in her ---- again!"

It took truly nimble footwork to keep ahead in this game. Unfortunately for all concerned, poor Mitzi seemed prone to recurring bouts of "hoo-hooitis!"

One of our most efficient and reliable receptionists was Peggy, who loved dogs and kept a stash of dog biscuits at her desk and in her purse for all her canine friends. One dog, dubbed "Hoggy" by the staff, was not content to wait for an appointment, but dropped by the hospital every morning for a handout. He would arrive about 11 a.m., which was feeding time for the hospital patients, and wait outside the front door until it was opened by an arriving or departing client. Seizing the moment, he would trot into the waiting room, jump onto a bench, and vault over the receptionist's counter. Tail wagging, he would turn his soulful eyes on Peggy and wait for his reward.

Hoggy lived some distance from the hospital, and eventually the inevitable happened — he was hit by a car on his way to visit us. We repaired his fractured hindleg, and he made a speedy recovery. Nothing daunted, he resumed his schedule of uninvited visits. Twice more he was hit by cars, but neither incident resulted in much damage (to Hoggy).

However, it was clear to the owners and to us that unless we forcefully discouraged him, he would eventually be killed or cause a serious automobile accident. He was adept at scaling fences, and no one could bear the thought of chaining him up all day. So Peggy and the rest of the staff steeled themselves to scold Hoggy, and resist his wiles. It took time, and some whacks with a rolled-up newspaper, but he eventually ceased to include our hospital in his appointed rounds.

Another of our receptionists was Carolyn. One day she brought in her fluffy new kitten, "Agnes," which she had gotten from a litter offered outside the supermarket. One of my colleagues gave Agnes her routine immunizations, and later, deworming medication. Almost everyone on the staff played with the kitten on its visits.

When the cat was nine months old, Carolyn asked me to spay Agnes. On the scheduled day, we anesthetized the cat, and Cheryl, the surgical nurse, shaved and scrubbed Agnes' belly. The cat was draped and placed on the operating table, and I donned my surgical garb.

I made the usual abdominal incision and began my unhurried search for the ovaries and uterus, just as I have done in thousands of other cats. Not finding them, I lengthened the incision and made another thorough search. I knew there had been no previous surgery; Carolyn had gotten Agnes as a kitten, and there was no scar.

Suddenly, it dawned on me. There is among veterinarians an ignominious fraternity — Veterinarians Who Have Spayed Tom Cats. It has happened to many a competent surgeon, and I had been warned about it by veterans. I had hoped never to join their ranks!

I put down my instruments in resignation. "Fold back the drapes and look under her tail," I said to Cheryl.

"Yep, he's got 'em," she replied sheepishly. She shared in the ignominy, since in the process of prepping the cat for surgery she should have checked for the presence of testicles.

I uttered an expletive or two, followed by a roar for Carolyn to present herself.

"We have a serious problem here," I said gravely as she stood in the doorway. "You're going to have to find a new name for your cat. 'Agnes' just doesn't make it for a tomcat!"

We all enjoyed that particular goof, since at least six of us should have ascertained the cat's sex by the time he reached nine months of age. Thereafter, all spay candidates were carefully scrutinized, and "Agnes" became known as "Angus."

Our night attendant was Johnny, a white-haired, one-armed Scotsman, with twinkling blue eyes and a love of animals. Although his right arm had been severed at the elbow in an industrial accident, he was able to accomplish more than many people with two hands. He would polish the floors till they shone, and make sure the animals' bedding was warm and dry. This was always accompanied by a behind-the-ears scratch and some kind words in his rich Scottish burr. I am sure that Johnny's care contributed to our patients' swift recoveries. Johnny was also a wonderful gardener, and supplied the waiting room and exam rooms with bouquets from his own garden.

When one of us was called in on a night-time emergency, Johnny was there to help. Some of my fondest memories are of sitting over tea and homemade scones with Johnny after an emergency case had been taken care of.

Late one evening I had a call from Johnny.

"Doctorrr Frrrye, Charrrlie has got himself into more than a wee bit of mischief this evening. He's let himself oot of his cage, and he's gone and opened the cages of the dogs and cats and yon two burrrds in the warrrd. Ye'd best hurry on doon."

Charlie was a young monkey who had been given to me, and who had become a hospital mascot. We had rigged up a large stainless steel cage for him, with swings and perches. He was immediately popular, and soon spoiled rotten.

When I arrived at the hospital that night, I opened the door of the ward on utter pandemonium. Charlie was swinging from the ceiling light fixture, looking down with delight on the scene he had created: dogs were chasing cats who were chasing birds and trying to elude the dogs! Bedlam!

Johnny and I worked for an hour corralling the rioters and getting them back in their respective cages. Amazingly, there were no casualties. We put a padlock on Charlie's cage, and the very next day a new home was found for him. The barter system works: I traded the mischief-maker for a new ten-speed bike!

Another hospital mascot was Samantha, an adult spayed female ocelot. She was given to me by a client who could no longer keep her in her apartment. Samantha was quite tame, and was let out of her cage at night to exercise in one of the wards. She had one game that was carefully explained to new employees and visitors: she liked to hide around blind corners and "attack." Fortunately, she never bit hard enough to cause injury.

One night Johnny phoned.

"Doctorrr Frrrye, it's aboot Sah-mahn-thah. When she was in the warrrd, she took a fancy to yon Afghan Hoond — the show dog. She's gone and been licking at its furrr."

"Johnny, don't worry, the fur will dry. Just put Samantha back in her cage," I said.

"But Doctorrr Frrrye, you don't understahnd. Therrre's more than a wee bit of furrr gone!"

I dressed in a hurry and drove to the hospital, fully expecting to see the makings of a monumental lawsuit. Indeed, a swathe of bare pink skin about three inches wide now ran the whole length of the hound, from the top of her head to the base of her elegant tail. Fortunately, the ocelot had not bitten the sleeping dog. Thank goodness for small favors! She had, however, put the Afghan out of the dog show circuit for some months to come.

Taking a deep breath, I dialed the owner.

"Hello, this is Dr. Frye. I'm calling because I'm concerned that Scheherezade has lost some hair from her back, upon awakening from her anesthesia," I said blandly.

"Oh doctor, how thoughtful of you to call. It's so late at night, and you're still caring for Scheherezade," she gushed. "Don't worry about her hair loss. I know it will grow back because once before when she stayed at another veterinary hospital, she came home missing some fur."

The next morning the woman came to retrieve her dog, and was not the least concerned by the reverse Mohawk hairdo. However, I'm sure that had I not called her the night before, all hell would have broken loose.

Now, I never will know what happened at that other hospital, but I am willing to wager that it was not associated with overzealous grooming by a pet ocelot's prickly tongue!

Almost every veterinarian has awakened in a cold sweat from the nightmare in which some calamity has befallen his practice or one of his or her patients. The fantasy is bad enough; the reality adds ten years to your age.

The trouble started when we agreed to board a particularly bad-tempered Miniature Poodle named "Go-Go" Green. His owners were going on vacation. Go-Go had been with us for a week or so when Stan, one of our aides, thinking the dog might like some sunshine, put him in the service yard where the refuse dumpster and oxygen tanks were located. Unfortunately, he forgot that it was Tuesday, the day that the gate out to the parking lot was left unlocked and ajar for the garbage collector.

The obvious happened: Go-Go went-went! A hastily recruited posse searched the neighborhood, calling his name and peering into every conceivable hidey-hole, with no success.

What could be worse?

Two hours later we had a call from the Berkeley Humane Society, saying that they had found a Miniature Poodle wearing one of our rabies tags. It was Go-Go! Much relieved, I said an aide would come immediately to retrieve the fugitive. The caller then demurred, "Well, there are some problems that will have to be dealt with."

"What kind of problems?" I asked cautiously.

"Sorry to have to tell you this, Doc, but the dog was apparently hit by a car."

"Is he alive?" I asked, fear gnawing at my belly.

"Sure, Doc, but he does have a few dings and dents." The voice was all too cheerful.

What could be worse?

"Look, Doc, there's one more problem with this little dog. It seems that when the driver went over to pick him up, the little bugger bit him."

What could be worse?

Go-Go had not only escaped, been hit by a car, and incarcerated in another establishment, but he was now under a ten-day rabies quarantine.

True to his tiny but wholly malicious nature, that damned dog had probably just *waited* until the Good Samaritan's hand was within range, then bit with glee!

We bailed Go-Go out, agreeing to observe the quarantine period. We spent over two hours cleansing and stitching his several lacerations, trying to make him presentable for his owners.

During this procedure, the hapless Stan who had put Go-Go in the yard hesitantly approached the surgery table, expecting to be dismissed. I was busy thinking of just *what* I was going to tell the Poodle's owners. As our young intern later related it, I was totally silent for a long time. Finally, after what must have seemed an eternity to Stan, I looked up, and fixing him with a mirthless gaze said quietly, "Stan, don't just stand there, place your scrotum on the table and surrender yourself to swift and sure justice!"

After that, the tension was gone. Go-Go made an uneventful recovery, and Stan is still working at the hospital. It is to the everlasting credit of the Greens that they accepted with equanimity my recounting of the terrible chain of events. I continued to see Go-Go until the time of my retirement from practice, though — perhaps understandably — he never mellowed towards any of us.

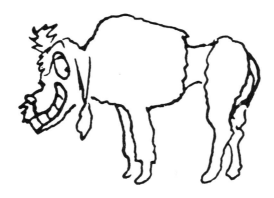

3 | Snakes and Snails and Puppy Dogs' Tails

I was an only child for the first five years of my life, born during the Great Depression. For some reason, I did not begin to speak until I was more than four years old. Because I was unusually tall for my age, this "handicap" seemed magnified. My parents recall the day when we all went for a special treat to the corner ice cream parlor in West Los Angeles where we lived. When asked by the counter girl what flavor I wanted, my reply was:

"Pah ba la ba la gum."

Looking at this otherwise normal, tall four-year-old uttering strange sounds, the woman clucked her tongue and shook her head — much to my parents' distress. *They* knew what I wanted: "Pineapple ice cream."

Shortly thereafter, I began to speak normally — in complete sentences and with a large vocabulary, much to the relief of my family.

In 1969 I was the recipient of the American Veterinary Medical Association's "Practitioner Research Award." I received the award at the AVMA annual meeting in Minneapolis. In separate telegrams to my parents, I wired "Pah ba la ba la gum. Love, Fred." Its meaning this time was clear to everyone, except the Western Union telegraphers and the clerk to whom I dictated it!

When I was five years old, my sister Susan was born. On the day she and my mother were to come home from the hospital, I was playing outside our apartment with "Keetah," a sleek Cocker Spaniel belonging to our landlord.

"Well Fred," said Mr. Walker, the landlord, "I guess you're excited to see your new baby sister."

I shrugged and stroked Keetah.

"Maybe you'd rather have a dog than a new baby sister," the old gentleman suggested slyly.

I looked up eagerly.

"I'll tell you what," said Mr. Walker, "how about a trade? I'll give you Keetah, and you give me the new baby?"

"Sure!" I said eagerly, reaching down for Keetah with excited hands.

Just then my father came out the door, car keys in hand.

"Well listen to this, Ben," said Mr. Walker. "Fred here is willing to trade me the new baby for Keetah. What do you say?"

My father looked from Mr. Walker to me, and back again. "Well, let's not complete the deal till you've both seen Susan," he said with a wink at Mr. Walker. "I'll be back in about an hour."

Keetah and I kept each other company peacefully until the battered Dodge sedan pulled up to the curb. My father leaped out and opened the door for my mother. She stood up, and folded back the blanket from my baby sister's face, for me to see.

I took one swift look at that small red face, and turned back to Keetah with an air of proprietorship. "Come on, Keetah," I said. "Let's go."

Mr. Walker and my parents looked at each other with amusement and some consternation. What to do? Mr. Walker came up with the solution: it would be Keetah who would go back on the deal. Everyone else was willing, I was told, but old Keetah would not agree to the trade. What could I say? Susan stayed with us, and I saw Keetah every day, but our relationship was never the same after *he* went back on our deal!

From the very beginning I was interested in animals, and especially reptiles. My mother was wonderfully tolerant of my interest, and often would drive me out into the Southern California desert to observe and collect animals. She would sit quietly reading in the oppressive heat while I climbed rock outcroppings and investigated dry stream beds, turning over flat rocks in search of lizards and other creatures. The fallen limbs of Joshua trees were always a likely hiding place for small snakes, centipedes, scorpions, spiders, and the live-bearing desert night lizard. Taking a canteen with me, I would spend several hours working a circular pattern around our car, and never become lost. I would come back for lunch, then go out again for another hour or two of scouring the desert floor.

My mother once returned from a vacation at a desert resort with a horned lizard, given to her by the hotel gardener. Then for my tenth birthday, my aunt gave me a baby boa constrictor. Before long, I was managing my own well-stocked menagerie.

My mother always insisted that my animals be fed, watered, and cleaned before I was fed. This was a splendid rule, and I never forgot what it meant to be responsible for the lives of others.

Years later, I came across the following passage from Antoine de Saint Exupery (1900-1944) which so aptly expresses what my mother wished to convey to me:

But if you tame me, then we shall need each other.
To me, you will be unique in all the world.
To you, I shall be unique in all the world.
You become responsible, forever, for what you have tamed. *

The staple diet of my snakes was mice. These could be bought at the local pet shop, but since I had a constant problem with cash flow, I was always looking for alternatives.

One day I heard on the herpetological grapevine that a nearby diagnostic lab would be giving away surplus mice that had been used in non-lethal experiments. All one had to do was show up on the specific days with a container, and pick up FREE mice!

On the appointed day, I took the bus to the lab, where I received twelve mice. Their appearance was striking. They had once been all white, but now were polka-dotted with spots of bright pink Merthiolate — presumably the sites of injections. I stowed this scurrying, motley crew in the cardboard cake box I had brought, and returned happily home.

We were living in the Los Feliz area of the Hollywood Hills at that time, and the walk from the bus stop to home was a hot one that day. Back at home I put the box of mice in the shade on the deck over our carport.

A few hours later, as we were sitting down to lunch, we heard loud screams from the house next door, the home of the actor Gene Lockhart. My first thought was that one of my snakes had escaped. But no — it was the forgotten mice, who had gnawed their way to freedom and traveled single-file down a vine-covered trellis, along a low stone wall, and through an open window into the Lockhart home. A servant had watched stupefied as twelve polka-dotted mice marched through the open window!

---

*The Little Prince, by Antoine de St. Exupery.

Rushing to the scene of the crime, my father and cousin and I spent twenty minutes scrambling around the Lockharts' well-appointed dining room, rounding up the fugitives.

Later, when we moved down to Hauser Boulevard, I hit on another idea for supplying my snakes with mice. I studied the mouse-traps at the hardware store, and decided to invest in three of them. A one-time outlay of cash, and then I would be supplied for life. But where to set them?

My mother would not let me insult our neighbors by asking if I could trap their mice. (Ours was a *respectable* neighborhood — one did not suspect his neighbors of having mice!) So I decided to turn my attention to the business district. There were two delicatessens and three bakeries within striking distance — surely a rich source of mice and rats!

Carrying my traps and a jar of peanut butter in a paper bag, I entered the swinging doors of the Wilshire Deli. The wooden floor was carpeted with sawdust, and the air fragrant with the mingled smells of spices, smoked meats, and cheeses. A haven for hungry rodents! A large woman was behind the cash register, reading a newspaper.

I cleared my throat. "I was wondering if I could trap some mice."

The woman stared at me, dumbfounded. "What did you say?" she said finally.

I held out one of my mousetraps. "I was wondering if I could trap some mice here," I repeated. "I need them to feed to my pet snakes."

The woman's eyes nearly popped. "Mice! We don't have any mice here. This place is spic and span! Inspected by the Health Department. Mice!" She picked up the newspaper and blocked me from her view.

Only slightly daunted, I continued on to Tony's Bakery, Hanne's Sandwich Shop, and the Good Times Liquor & Deli. At each it was the same story: a huffy denial that they ever *had* mice. Mice? It was as though I were asking if they had leprosy.

Finally, at the Cottage Bakery, I struck pay dirt. Yes, they had mice, and the health department would not allow them to keep a cat. I was ushered into the fragrant kitchen like a welcomed guest.

Under the gaze of two bakers who had paused in their rolling and patting, I lined up my traps and baited them with peanut butter. This, I knew, was irresistible to mice, even more so than cheese. I placed the traps at strategic points in the pantry storeroom: on the floor behind the bins of flour, on a shelf near some sacks of sugar, and one in the corner behind the door. I left certain of success.

This was the beginning of a long and happy relationship. Not only did I come away each day with a discreet paper bag of dead mice for my snakes in one hand, but always in the other was a square of dark semisweet chocolate for me — a gift of the grateful bakers. (In those World War II days, chocolate was hard to come by, and a distinct luxury.)

When I was ten, my mother and sister went on a three-week visit to relatives in Toronto. (I was supposed to go too, but protested adamantly that I would *not* wear scratchy wool trousers. My mother capitulated and let me stay home with my father.) My mother and Susan had no sooner left Los Angeles than I converted my bedroom into a veritable jungle setting, complete with several aquaria full of frogs, toads, and newts, some cages of snakes, a caged bat, and jars of spiders and scorpions. (In the 1940's it was not yet known that bats are hosts and transmitters of wild-life rabies.)

I belonged to a Junior Explorer Club and with them had made several trips down to Seal Beach to a seedy roadside snake emporium. Hand-painted signs along the roadside whetted one's appetite long before the ramshackle collection of sheds came into view: "See the deadly cobras!" "See the man-eating alligators!" "Six-foot rattlers!"

The establishment was run by two old ladies: Miss Grace Olive Wiley, a well-known semi-professional herpetologist, and her wizened mother. They lived together in a battered trailer adjacent to the animal sheds.

Miss Wiley would put on little reptile "shows," handling the deadly snakes herself. In me she sensed a kindred spirit, and we made several trades of specimens.

While my mother was in Toronto, I persuaded my father to drive me down to the reptile emporium. Seal Beach was an hour and a half by car from our home, and gas was rationed, so such an expedition was a rare treat. I have forgotten by now what specimens I took to trade, but I came away with a five-and-a-half-foot American Alligator named Pokey.

Imagine my joy! My father and I got Pokey into the trunk of the car, and drove home. It was winter, and even in Los Angeles, too cold for the alligator to live outdoors. Naturally, I installed him in my room, where he spent most of his time under the bed. My adjoining bathroom shower was convenient for bathing him.

In our communications with my mother in Toronto, my father and I diplomatically made no mention of the latest addition to the household. It would be a nice surprise when she got home.

The three weeks flew by, and my father and I picked up my mother and Susan at the airport. On the way home I endured Susan's raptures about the snow, about the people they had met, about the plane trip.

"Mother, I want to show you something in my room," I said, as soon as we were in the house.

I opened the door, and my mother had her first sight of the jungle transformation. Pokey was out of sight under the bed.

"Oh Fred, what have you done?" said my mother in dismay, sinking down on the bed. Immediately there was a loud hiss, and Pokey's snout emerged between her ankles.

Drawing herself up onto the bed, my mother kept her usual calm, until the alligator had crawled to the center of the room.

"All right, Fred," she said evenly, "I want that animal out of my house. O-U-T. And I—mean—NOW!"

I went into my tale about the cold nights, and she finally relented for that one night, as long as Pokey was shut in the bathroom. But the next day when I returned from school I found a truck parked in the driveway, and two men busily remodeling my sister's playhouse into an alligator habitat. When completed, it had a cement wading pool and was securely enclosed by a chainlink fence.

Pokey was quite tame, and would allow me to haul him out onto the back lawn without any protest. He continued to grow, and by the time I was in junior high school, he was almost seven feet long, and weighed about ninety pounds.

At that time, one of my favorite teachers asked me to bring my alligator for Open House Night. On that Friday night, my father and I drove Pokey to school, where we placed him in the classroom behind a barricade of table tops propped up with chairs. I was to remain with him during the evening's festivities. I swelled with pride as the first group of my classmates and their parents approached.

"Hey guys — look at the crocodile!"

"Yah! Sssssss!"

They leaned over the table tops, snapping their fingers and hissing. Pokey regarded them balefully.

"He's not a crocodile, he's an American alligator. Crocodiles have thinner heads and longer noses," I said. "Don't tease him, you might upset him."

"Hey Fred — does he bite? Man, look at those teeth!"

"What does he eat? Would he eat this eraser? Let's see what he does with it!"

"Please leave him alone," I repeated, sensing Pokey's growing agitation.

"Hey look at this!" said one large boy, dangling a string in front of the reptile's nose.

Pokey uttered a loud hiss and made an open-mouthed rush at the arms hanging over his barricade. The girls squealed in terror, and the boys roared in delight.

I leaned over the barricade and tried to talk soothingly, but Pokey thrashed his tail and hissed. He was a totally different creature from the tame pet I knew. But then, this was his first experience of teasing. Miss Wiley had raised him with love and care, and I, too, had always been gentle with him.

The Open House was due to end at 9 p.m., and never had the hands on the schoolroom clock moved so slowly. Finally, at 9:15, the last stragglers had gone, and my parents and Mr. Conway and I stood and looked at Pokey. He still thrashed his tail and hissed whenever I approached, and we decided to leave him where he was overnight. A reluctant janitor agreed to meet us at school the next morning.

The next day I recruited my friend Don to help me maneuver Pokey. My father was willing to chauffeur us in his convertible, but not to participate in any alligator wrestling. Happily, there was no wrestling involved. Pokey was back to his calm self, and we just pick-

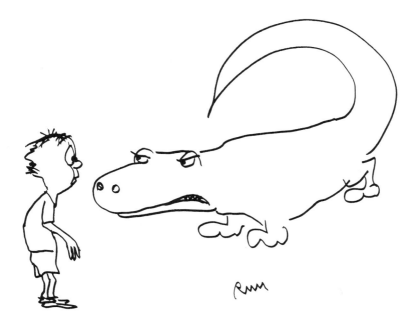

ed him up like a limber log. The janitor saw us to the door with undisguised relief.

We had planned to put Pokey in the trunk, but Don and I persuaded my father to let us keep him with us in the back seat. It was such a beautiful warm day, and poor Pokey had not had any fresh air since the day before. He *deserved* a treat, to make up for last night's bad experiences.

We set out for home, the sun shining down in our faces, the wind rushing by our ears. Suddenly we were aware of honking behind us, and of people pointing frantically at the back of the car. Pokey was perched on the trunk of the convertible.

My father stepped on the brakes, and the alligator slid down the trunk, bounced against the bumper, and hit the street with a slap. He was instantly enraged, hissing, thrashing his tail, and snapping his tooth-studded jaws.

We were on a busy street through a residential area, and nearby a gardener was watering flower beds with a hose. My father borrowed this, and I turned it on Pokey while goggle-eyed motorists threaded their way past us. Two police officers arrived, and asked my father some uncomfortable questions. Don and I held the hose and watched silently as one of the officers slowly filled out several ominous-looking papers.

Finally Pokey was cooled down enough to be picked up. Wordlessly, my father opened the trunk, and Don and I put the alligator inside. My father shut the lid, and locked it for good measure.

Back in the car, instead of continuing on home, my father swung around and headed for the road to Seal Beach. This had been the last straw — Pokey had to return to Miss Wiley's reptile emporium. I pleaded Pokey's case all the way, but with the sinking feeling that it was to no avail.

When we arrived at the familiar collection of sheds with corrugated tin roofs, Miss Wiley was being interviewed by the well-known free-lance writer, Dan Mannix, and photographed handling some deadly cobras. She interrupted the session to graciously accept the alligator back. Pokey was put in a pen with two smaller crocodilians, a pair of bad-tempered South American spectacled caimans.

We drove towards home in silence, interrupted only when my father turned on the car radio. A few minutes later we heard a news flash that Miss Grace Olive Wiley, well-known amateur herpetologist, had been bitten by a cobra she was handling, and had been rushed to the hospital. She died less than an hour later.

So I lost Pokey and an old friend, and Pokey lost me and his "Mother" all on the same day.

I still had a large menagerie to console me. My collection had long since outgrown my bedroom, and now was housed in the garage, displacing the two family cars. I had two large floor-to-ceiling aviary-type cages housing a pink-eyed albino opossum and her normal-colored would-be mate (with whom she would have nothing to do), and a female Texas nine-banded armadillo.

Hanging from the open rafters were two cylindrical cages holding inverted, sleeping bats.

On the floor, large galvanized washtubs partially filled with water contained assorted turtles and two young caimans (alligator-like animals from South America).

On shelves were about twenty-four glass-fronted snake and lizard cages, each illuminated by a small incandescent bulb.

On another wall was the food supply for many of these: small cages of rats, mice and hamsters, which I now bred and sometimes traded for equipment or animals at a couple of pet shops. No more laboratory cast-offs!

In one corner were a number of aquaria filled with tadpoles, newts, toads and frogs.

The atmosphere in the garage was tolerable since I cleaned all cages regularly, and only the opossums, rodents, bats and armadillo produced much odor.

In retrospect, I appreciate how very tolerant my parents were of my hobby. My mother only drew the line at monkeys and parrots. Armadillos, snakes, lizards — yes; monkeys and parrots — no.

As my menagerie grew, feeding them took more and more of my spare time. My bats and lizards ate grasshoppers and crickets, and I became adept at catching these in the vacant lots near our home. My system with crickets was quite simple: I cut apart cardboard cartons, and distributed the flat pieces of cardboard around the vacant lot. A few days later, I had only to bring my jar and make the rounds of my "cricket apartments." The insects made their homes under the cardboard, and I could readily harvest them.

I also spent time digging for earthworms and gathering slugs in our backyard — my turtles and birds (at various times a shrike, a sparrow hawk, a screech owl and a raven) devoured these, as did the lizards, armadillo, and moles and shrews. (A shrew will eat its own weight in food every day, and so I was kept busy!) Later, I raised mealworms in trays of bran. (The owl and hawk also ate mice and large insects.)

Moths were another delicacy for the lizards and bats, and I had two sources for them. There were many flowering lantana bushes in the yards up and down Hauser Boulevard where we lived, and these are especially attractive to butterflies and moths.

A more exciting source was to go in the evening several blocks to where an appliance store featured in its window two or three of those current novelties, televisions. The bluish light emanating from the black-and-white TV screens attracted moths to the plate glass window, where they could be plucked off. My sister Susan often accompanied me on these forays. The challenge lay in getting more moths *into* our paper bags without letting the rest *out*.

Beef heart is highly recommended as an occasional treat for turtles. By returning empty soda bottles for their meager deposit, and doing odd jobs, I was able to sometimes buy this delicacy for my creatures. On one occasion I got some for free, but it was not worth the price I paid in youthful embarrassment.

I stood at the meat counter of the local grocery, my change making a comfortable weight in my jeans pocket. Around me, other customers were selecting Sunday dinner roasts and packages of ground beef.

My turn came, and I looked up into the round, florid face of the butcher and said, "I'd like some beef hearts, please."

The butcher smiled broadly and turned to his cohort who was weighing out some bacon. "Did you hear that?" he said loudly. "The lad says he wants some bee farts."

I felt myself growing very hot, and stared straight ahead at the coils of sausage decorated with parsley. After an eternity, in which I wondered how many customers were staring at me, a great red hand slapped a white package in front of me.

"There you go, son."

I fumbled in my pocket, but the jovial voice said, "No charge, son. I had some extra." Obviously, he was feeling some remorse. Mumbling my thanks, I clutched the package and fled.

I remember the day when my father squared himself up for the unwelcome task of having a "birds and bees" talk with his growing son. Both of my parents were quite "modern" in their outlook, but when it came to discussing sex with one of his own children, my father was not in his best form.

He began circuitously, and soon became so entangled in his own explanations that he stopped, at a loss as to how to proceed. But I had begun to grasp what this strange conversation was about.

"Oh, you mean sex," I said. "Heck, I've known how animals mate and reproduce for years! Come out to the garage with me."

He looked at me dubiously, but with some relief. "What's so special out there?" he asked.

"Oh, nothing new to me, but it's something you might like to see," I said.

Earlier that morning, I had noticed that one of my female hamsters was in heat. Ushering my father into the garage, I took down her cage and one containing a male hamster. As soon as the two were together in the male's cage, he began to sniff and court the receptive female. In a few moments, they were copulating.

My father watched this procedure with some discomfiture. When he had regained some of his poise, he asked me a few questions about the reproductive cycle in hamsters.

That was the end of our "birds and bees" conversation — surely one of the most illuminating ever held between a father and his son!

Across the street from us on Hauser Boulevard was the home of the actor Don DeFore. We often saw him on weekends, assiduously manicuring his front lawn. The houses on that side of the street were built at a slightly higher elevation than on ours, and Don DeFore's lawn was a putting-green perfect slope from the house to the street.

No sooner would an airborne dandelion seed germinate and emerge among the Kentucky bluegrass, than Mr. DeFore would be on his knees extracting it. After such an exercise, he would cross over to our side of the street and stand looking back lovingly at his verdant turf.

One day I gave a tour of my menagerie to a visiting friend of my mother's from Canada. At the end of it, she asked if she could actually handle a snake. With great pride, I selected an eight-foot boa constrictor and carried it out to the front lawn.

I draped the docile, vibrantly colored snake around the woman's shoulders. She seemed to enjoy the experience, and my mother took several snapshots. As a grand finale, the snake coiled its entire length around the woman's torso.

We were uncoiling it — I holding the snake near the head, the woman gently turning around and around — when a pre-war luxurious LaSalle sedan came up the street. Seeing an eight-foot snake suspended between a woman and a young boy, the driver kept her startled eyes on us, and the huge car drifted toward our side of the street. Recalled to her driving, the woman swung the wheel wildly in the other direction — toward Don DeFore's prized lawn!

The car struck the curb with a shriek of tortured metal, mowed down a tree, and careened up the slope. It teetered at an angle for a moment, then slid sideways down the incline, until stopped by the fallen tree. It rested there like a great, beached whale.

We rushed to the scene. The two women occupants of the car were shaken but unhurt. The car had sustained considerable damage to its front end, and a tow truck was called. But the greatest casualty was Don DeFore's lawn. The green slope was scarred by tire-excavated furrows, and great swathes of turf had been scraped off by the side-slipping automobile, exposing the soil and the underground sprinkler system.

The police officer called to this scene of botanical carnage listened politely to the woman driver's tale of woe. Then, as she waited for the tow truck, he walked over to our house to see for himself the proximate cause of the accident.

As it turned out, he was a World War II veteran and part-time student of zoology at Los Angeles City College. I gave him a complete tour of my menagerie, and he chatted amicably with my mother, praising the quality and health of my animal collection. Thus any threat to my "zoo" as a public nuisance was nipped in the bud.

However, there was still Mr. DeFore to be faced. He was away at the movie studio, and I watched for his return with a feeling of dread.

From our living room window I saw his car turn into their driveway and stop. There was a long pause, and then Mr. DeFore emerged slowly, like a man in a daze. His wife appeared and began gesturing — at the street, at our house, at the broken tree and the lawn.

My parents sent me across the street to apologize for my part in the affair. After the initial shock, Don DeFore accepted the situation with good grace, and was even able to see the humor in it. I promised never again to display any of my unusual creatures in front of our house.

When I was in junior high school, one of my best friends was Jason Albertson, whose father managed a movie theater on Wilshire Boulevard. Jason and I could always get into the *El Rey* for free, and we availed ourselves of this privilege nearly every weekend. Ensconced in the red plush seats, we enjoyed such thrillers as "The Phantom of the Opera," "Frankenstein," and "The Picture of Dorian Gray."

However, we soon hit on a plan to augment the terror of these spine chillers. While other people carried bags of popcorn to their seats, we sat in the back row with bags of a different sort. Fluttering around inside was last night's haul of moths. At the appropriate moment, we would release these, and the flying insects would head for the lights, wreaking havoc on the screen. A moth with a one-inch wing span would be magnified into a six-foot flying monster as it closed in on the projection lamp.

Fortunately for us, Jason's father was a laid-back, mellow guy. Although there were a few screams, and a few fastidious people left in disgust, the movie rolled on uninterrupted. Jason and I slouched gleefully in our seats.

The high point of our movie career was when we smuggled in a bag containing two bats, as well as the now-standard bag of moths. The movie was "The Picture of Dorian Gray." Waiting until the peak of terror, we released first the moths, who headed for the projector's beam.

"I'll count to twenty, then I'll let the bats go," I whispered to Jason, under cover of the general stir from the audience.

". . . seventeen, eighteen, nineteen, twenty!" The bats flew free of the bag, and headed in hot pursuit of the moths, their natural prey.

Cries went up from the audience as the bats' silhouettes crossed the screen. Like the moths, they were hugely magnified, till they looked like enormous winged beasts from the age of the dinosaurs.

"Look at that! Look at that!" I said exultantly to Jason. "They look just like pterodactyls!"

The audience continued to shriek and cower, as though the theatre were indeed invaded by those prehistoric flying reptiles.

One of the huge beasts captured its prey and swallowed it, as the audience gasped in horror.

Jason and I were in ecstasies. A few persons fled past us in the aisles, and we heard Jason's father in the lobby, giving reassurances that there was no danger.

"Imagine!" I chortled. "Attacked by a moth!"

"This is the greatest!" Jason repeated for the tenth time. "We'll never top this!"

And he was right. Looking back, I can see that this was the absolute pinnacle of our career in movie sabotage!

A favorite visitor to our home was Harry, a salesman who worked for my father. He was middle-aged, unmarried, and talked with a

Brooklyn accent that delighted Susan and me. His last name was Wolff, and she and I called him, with great affection, "Mr. Howl."

One Sunday afternoon when Harry was invited for supper, I gave him a tour of my menagerie. It was a balmy spring day, with the sweet scent of blossoms wafting on the breezes. A pair of western bullsnakes had chosen that afternoon to complete their courtship and commence their prolonged copulation.

"You're lucky today," I said to Harry. "Look at this. They're just beginning to mate."

Harry looked from me to the scene inside the glass snake cage, and stood frozen. The male snake was lying alongside the female, and was preparing to copulate.

What few non-herpetologists know (and certainly unknown to innocent bachelor Harry) is that male snakes have a *pair* of external sex organs, which they use alternately during copulations. These are located side by side, a few centimeters apart, low on the snake's body. They are usually withdrawn, and so are not normally seen.

Now, however, everything was in full view, under the embarrassed and fascinated gaze of Harry.

"They'll keep that up for as long as twenty-four hours," I said cheerfully.

Harry said nothing, but continued to gaze at the intent activity in the glass cage.

"Now over here I have my opossums. This is the female, but she won't let the male mate with her . . ." Harry followed me wordlessly, as I continued the tour of my collection.

That night at dinner, Harry was unusually silent. Susan and I withdrew after the dessert, and later when I passed the living room, I heard Harry's earnest voice.

"Ben! Ann! I could not *believe* the things that young Fred showed me this afternoon. I'm telling you, I was shocked! How can you allow him access to such things? It's not suitable for a young boy. Those snakes--" He stopped, at a loss for words.

I continued on to my bedroom. But the rise and fall of Harry's voice continued for a long time afterwards.

I continued to see Harry after I grew up, and to his dying day he remembered those amorous bullsnakes. Further, he never wavered in his conviction that my parents were wrong in allowing me to have such a *perverted* hobby!

4 | More Confessions of an Incorrigible Animal Fancier

I stood at attention as the executive officer worked his way down the row of lockers. Since my arrival at the U.S. Naval Air Facility at Norman, Oklahoma, such "snap" inspections had often yielded contraband food, beer, or hard liquor. (Oklahoma was officially a "dry" state in 1952, although several local gas stations dispensed high-test potables in their back rooms. One audacious owner actually had a gas pump hooked to a tank of moonshine whiskey. It was an old-fashioned pump with a high glass cylinder, in which a propeller spun as the golden-brown fluid was pumped out. Strictly high octane material!)

The executive officer had found nothing yet in his random check, and now was stopped in front of my locker. I stared straight ahead and willed him to pass on. He opened the metal door and began feeling through the folded clothes. Suddenly he uttered a cry, and his hand recoiled as though he had received an electric shock.

"Damn," I thought to myself, "which one of my creatures bit him?"

He opened the metal door wider, revealing a small box turtle that had been sleeping in my watch cap.

"What's the meaning of this?" he roared.

"I'm studying him, sir. A biology project. I'm going to release him as soon as I get some time off."

"Hmm. Got anything else in there, Frye?" He was obviously reluctant to put his hand in again.

"Only a praying mantis, sir. In a glass jar. She's laying her eggs right now, and can't be disturbed." Best not to mention the bullsnake, I decided.

He looked at me, stupefied. Booze and ordinary contraband he could deal with; this was beyond his realm. Beyond the farthest reaches of the military code.

"All right, Frye," he said ominously, "present yourself in your dress blue uniform in my office in one hour."

An hour later, showered, shaved and uniformed, I stood at full-brace attention before this stern-faced naval officer. The stigma of court-martial kept intruding itself unwelcomely on my mind. What would my parents say?

"Here is a one-day pass, Frye. Now take your animals and go! And you'd better not return to this base with anything or anybody who hasn't taken the loyalty oath!"

Two hours later I deposited the turtle, the snake, and the mantis with her egg mass (by this time securely cemented to a twig) in the rural area beyond Oklahoma City where I'd found them.

This left me with the rest of the day free! I took in a movie, had a good meal, and returned to the barracks long after sundown. All thanks to my unauthorized collecting of animals.

I had joined the Navy straight out of high school — without completing high school, to tell the truth. But luckily for me, at that time (1952, the time of the Korean conflict), servicemen who scored well on aptitude tests were given the opportunity to take high school and college courses through the U.S. Armed Forces Institute (USAFI).

I was deemed one of the "educable" ones, and once I had completed basic training, I realized that performing well academically was the only alternative to endless marching, assignment to loathesome duty stations, or immediate shipment to the war zone. I signed up for as full a course load as I could manage, which included college biology from Yale University, and English from the University of California at Berkeley. I justified the military's investment in me by taking courses in military law, economics, and celestial navigation. (The Navy's interest was in developing potential instructors for its specialty schools; I eventually became an instructor of specialized aircraft welding.)

For an initial three-dollar fee, the USAFI supplied the textbooks and prepaid postage to and from the various participating universities. I corresponded with my instructors, and took proctored exams. After three years of active duty in the Navy, I had completed one and a half years' worth of college credit, all for that three-dollar investment!

I learned "Aviation Fundamentals" and "Aviation Structures" at the Navy School at Norman, Oklahoma. This included courses in aircraft welding, metalsmithing and machining. I studied aeronautics and aerostatics at the Ground and Flight School for blimps in Lakehurst, New Jersey.

Later I was assigned to an experimental blimp squadron at Key West, Florida. Our mission was to develop anti-submarine tactics. Between flights, we were free of duties for several days at a time. On one such day, I went out on a commercial sports fishing boat, in the Florida Straits.

The skipper of this craft was a one-eyed woman named Shirley, who could outswear and outdrink most men twice her size. She had lost an eye some time before, but refused to wear a glass eye. Instead, she wore dark glasses night and day to cover the loss.

After I had made a few excursions with Captain Shirley, she gruffly offered me a job as relief first mate on her boat. I had a lot of free time, and accepted.

Although it was nominally against the Florida Fish and Game regulations to sell game fish taken in state waters, Shirley had a commercial license to sell snapper, pompano and grouper to the local restaurant trade. She would take a full share of what we earned, and Raoul, the young Cuban deckhand, and I would split another share between us.

One day we picked up a party of businessmen in Miami, and headed out to the Florida Straits. Along the way, we stopped in proven fishing grounds to let the party try for giant grouper and sharks. Groupers weighing over two hundred pounds were not uncommon in the deep waters of this area, and soon one of the men had one on.

"Look at that! It's a two-hundred-pounder at least!" The others gathered around.

The pole was bent almost double; the taut line glistened in the sunlight. Suddenly it shuddered, and went slack.

"You lost him! You lost him! The hook must've worked itself free." There was a general sigh of disappointment. The angler continued to reel in his line, to inspect his hooks. A strange form took shape beneath the water and surfaced: the huge head of a grouper, hooks still in its jaws, and torn from its body just behind the gills.

"Would you look at that!" The party crowded around excitedly.

"A shark got it, sure as shooting."

"Man, what a shark that must've been!"

We all felt a tremor of frightened delight at the thought.

"Well, that baby would've been a two-hundred-pounder, no doubt about it," said one man consolingly as the angler laid the head on the deck and disentangled his hooks.

"Two-twenty, I'd say," said Shirley in her gravelly voice.

We looked at the giant head in awe, and tried to imagine what had happened there in the deep.

The men went back to their fishing with renewed energy, and in the next forty minutes two more bodyless groupers were reeled in. When this happened, shadowy forms were seen swimming around the boat. The businessmen were as excited as schoolboys. To lose a fish to a shark was far better than bringing one home. The tales they would have to tell!

"Time to move on," said Shirley eventually, and went into the wheelhouse. She started the engine, and the boat began backing. Suddenly there was a loud noise below, from the vicinity of the propellers.

"Hell!" said Shirley, and shut the engine down. "Sounds like I've backed her over the ----ing port anchor line."

Raoul and I looked over the side. It was true. Obviously, the rope was entangled in either the propeller or its shaft.

"Son of a bitch!" said Shirley. "Let's cut the ----ing line and see what happens."

We did so, but to no avail. The anchor line was inextricably wound around some part of the propeller mechanism.

"Well Hell," said our skipper. "We've either got to set here and wait for the ----ing Coast Guard, or someone's got to go under there and free that ----ing thing."

There was a pregnant silence, and Raoul and I exchanged glances. He looked at the horizon, and said nothing. The vacationing businessmen stood listening to this exchange with ill-suppressed excitement.

"I got my gun," said Shirley, pointing with her thumb toward the cabin. "I can cover you if you go over the side." The dark glasses looked at me inscrutably.

I thought of the crewman in our squadron back at Key West who had gone swimming and been killed by a barracuda. Not a pleasant way to die.

Still, at age nineteen most of us still believe ourselves to be immortal; we can not yet imagine that we could actually cease to be.

"Okay, I'll give it a try," I said, bending over to untie my shoes.

An excited murmur went up among our passengers. "Okay you guys," rasped Shirley, "You can take those gaff hooks and cover him from the side there. Raoul, you take my gun and get up on the roof of the wheelhouse."

I dove over the side, and came up alongside the large three-bladed propellers. As we had guessed, the nylon anchor line was wound around the shaft of one of these. My fingers went to work on the tangle and made some progress, and then I had to surface for air.

"Well, how bad is the bitch?" yelled Shirley from above.

"Not bad," I gasped. "I've almost got it."

"Okay," she said shortly, the sun glinting on her dark glasses.

I dove again, and my fingers again automatically did their job, while the rest of me was oblivious to time and space. The tangle came loose and fell away in my hands. I soared toward the sun, the air.

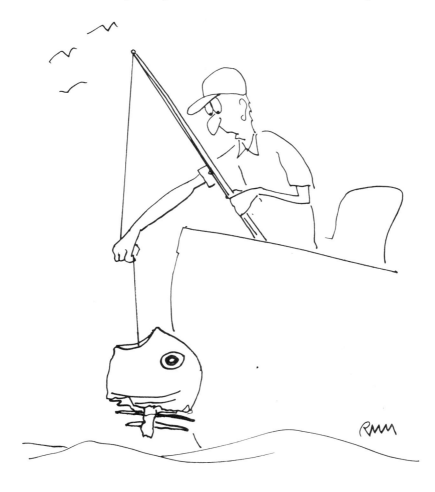

"How's it going?"

"Done," I gasped. I swam to the side, where a phalanx of rusty gaff hooks guarded my re-boarding. A half-dozen hands reached out to help me back on board.

"Good job!"

"Nice going!"

Slaps on the back, shakings of hands.

"Well, young man, we owe you a great deal," said a portly, gray-haired man in a Hawaiian shirt. He extracted his wallet from his pocket, and pulled out a twenty-dollar bill. "Here's a little tip, with my thanks."

"Thank you," I said, as the water streamed from my clothes, "but that's not necessary."

"No, no, I insist," said my determined benefactor. "What is your name, young man?"

"Fredric Frye, sir, Second Class Petty Officer, U.S. Navy."

"Well, Fred, if you need a job when you get out of the Navy, just let me know." And he handed me his business card. He was the chairman of a large corporation in New York.

"All right, Raoul, give me back that gun," yelled Shirley. "Lucky we didn't see any sharks, Fred. Raoul might've shot you instead!" She gave a short laugh. "Let's get going, let's get going. We gotta be back in Miami by five o'clock. And I sure as hell could use a drink."

When I completed my three years of active duty in the Navy, I returned to Los Angeles, and enrolled in pre-veterinary courses at Santa Monica City College. The classes were at night; in the daytime I supported myself by working as an advertising specialties salesman. I also apprenticed myself to a local veterinarian, Dr. James Wilson, who let me volunteer my services as kennel cleaner, performer of simple lab tests, and willing learner of all that could be absorbed from the everyday routine of a veterinary hospital.

I had never actually seen surgery performed, but the Pre-Med Club at UCLA showed free surgery movies on Friday evenings. I attended these eagerly. I stretched out my long limbs in the front row, and watched, rapt, as the deft, gloved hands performed all manner of procedures and maneuvers. The blood and internal organs didn't faze me; I felt I was ready for anything.

One day Dr. Wilson said, "Say, Fred, I'm planning to perform a new surgical technique next week. Something I heard about at a recent veterinary meeting, for devoicing dogs."

I looked up eagerly from the blood count I was doing.

"My clients the Goodmans have this Wire Haired Terrier that's driving the neighbors crazy with barking. They've complained to the police, and so now the choice is to get rid of the dog, or try this." He polished his glasses on his smock.

"The procedure doesn't seem too complicated, but I'll need a special instrument for it. You've told me that you were trained as a machinist in the Navy, and I was hoping you could construct what we need."

I was eager and confident, and over the next few days painstakingly designed and built on a borrowed lathe the prescribed tool. It was a long stainless steel device, with two cutting-edged cups at the end. The handle held a plunger. When this was depressed against an internal spring, the cups came together, and were capable of snipping out small circles of soft tissue. I polished the finished instrument lovingly, wrapped it in tissue paper, and proudly presented it to Dr. Wilson.

"Say, Fred, this looks first-rate," he said, flexing the plunger and watching the two cups snap together.

I smiled modestly.

"I'll tell you what. I'd like you to see it in action. Let's schedule the ventriculocordectomy for next Saturday afternoon, and you can assist me."

I could hardly wait for Saturday. It finally came, hot and humid. The terrier's barking echoed through the hospital as my mentor and I ate our lunches.

"Slow down, slow down," said Dr. Wilson kindly as I bolted the last of my sandwich and drained my carton of milk. "Old Buster might as well enjoy a last hearty bark. When we're done, he'll just sound like he's coughing, according to what I've heard. They don't seem to realize it, though, and go through all the motions, quite happily. Here, have some of my wife's brownies. She's got a family recipe that can't be beat."

I was already full, but accepted two brownies, and tried not to eat them too fast.

"Now then," said Dr. Wilson, standing up and brushing crumbs from his smock. "Let's see if old Buster is ready to pipe down."

This was in the mid-1950's, and modern anesthesia had yet to be introduced in veterinary medicine. We put Buster on the operating table, and covered his muzzle with a funnel-like mask holding a wad of cotton gauze, into which ether was dripped.

Since our surgical site was the larynx, below the muzzle, we had to remove the ether mask in order to proceed, and then reapply it whenever the anesthetic level seemed insufficient. In the course of these maneuvers, ether fumes wafted around us. (As I think back to these crude methods, I shudder. Ether fumes are highly inflammable; more than one surgical team and their patients have been killed or maimed by operating room accidents involving ether fumes.)

Nonetheless, I was fascinated by this my first experience of live surgery. I bent over the dog's open mouth, watching every move the surgeon made. With each snip of my untried instrument, the dog coughed great clouds of bloody mist, like a harpooned whale. This sprayed over my face and glasses, as I followed every move...

The next thing I knew, Dr. Wilson was dragging me out to the patio by the armpits.

"What happened?" I murmured, breathing in the warm fresh air and trying to focus my eyes behind the blood-spattered glasses.

"You passed out there, Fred," said Dr. Wilson, somewhat anxiously. "You feel all right now?"

"Yes, yes. Just let me sit here a minute."

"It's hot," said the doctor, pulling off his surgical mask and stripping off his rubber gloves. "I've never known it to be so humid in July."

I sat on the ground, breathing deeply.

"Well," he said kindly, "You're not the first person to pass out at the sight of blood. You should have seen yourself! You fell right across the table — just about pushed old Buster onto the floor. Instruments flying in all directions. I had a time of it getting you out here — you're no lightweight, my boy."

He teased me gently for a few more minutes about my squeamishness, and we went back in, got out some new sterile surgical packs, and completed the job.

Later, as I thought over this humiliating introduction to surgery, I was convinced that my downfall was due to the heat and humidity, the ether fumes, and my over-full stomach. Undone by Mrs. Wilson's homemade brownies!

Since that memorable July day, many changes have taken place. Firstly, anesthesia is now accomplished with closed-circuit machines using non-explosive anesthetic agents. Secondly, the proper instruments for ventriculocordectomy are readily available, and make the procedure practically bloodless. I have performed hundreds of these operations since I graduated from veterinary school and completed my surgical residency. Lastly, as a result of my own introduction to surgery, I have always been very sympathetic to anyone who has grown faint while watching *me* performing the surgeon's art!

I was living at home at this time, and dating my high school sweetheart. We had corresponded at fairly regular intervals while I was in the Navy. We both assumed that we would get married some day, but I was not in any hurry to rush into that blissful state.

One morning at breakfast my mother sprang some news on me.

"Fred, you know my friend Ceil Schwalb, don't you?"

I stirred my cereal and tried to bring my mind to bear on this heavy question.

"Yes, I guess I do," I agreed.

"Well, she has some Canadian relatives, the Kleins, who moved here a few months ago, from Vancouver, British Columbia." My mother had many relatives and connections in Canada; Canadians were always of interest to her.

"Oh."

"Well, Ceil was telling me yesterday that the Kleins' daughter has just arrived in town. She was studying abroad when her parents moved, and so is a total stranger here."

"Oh."

"So, I told Ceil that you would call her up, and invite her out to dinner some evening soon."

I dropped my spoon. "Mother! How can you do that? You know that Sandy and I are more or less going together. I don't need to get involved with any other girl. Besides, I can't afford to take anybody out to dinner right now." I picked up my spoon and stabbed the cereal.

"I'll pay, dear. I'll be happy to. Just this once — just invite her once, as a favor to me."

"You'll pay? God — she must be a real dog! Have you seen her?"

"No, dear, but I'm sure she's very nice. Her name is Brucye."

I finally relented and agreed to take this Canadian girl out — *just once.* "But I won't take your money," I said to my mother, holding out on this one point of honor.

"As you like, dear."

Then there was the awkward phone call to endure.

"Hello, is this Brucye Klein?"

"Yes it is." (A pleasant, musical voice.)

"Well, my name is Fred Frye. You don't know me," (such a hackneyed phrase, I thought, picking up speed) "but my mother is a friend of Mrs. Schwalb, who is a friend of your parents." A pause for breath.

"Oh. I see."

"And so, I was calling to see if you'd like to go out to dinner on Saturday night." (What an idiot — why should she want to go out to dinner with a complete stranger?)

"Well, that sounds very nice. Yes, I would like to."

At 6:30 on Saturday night, I knocked on the Kleins' door. It was opened by a small, older woman — Mrs. Klein, I safely guessed.

"Fred? Hello, I'm Mrs. Klein. Just a minute, I'll go call Brucye."

I stood in the hall, not wanting to have to make small talk with Mr. Klein, who no doubt was lurking in the living room. I was regretting having consented to this ordeal.

Mrs. Klein returned with her daughter, a lovely slender blonde girl, taller than her mother, who smiled and held out her hand.

"Fred? Hello, I'm Brucye. This is nice of you to befriend a new person in town."

My favorable first impression increased as the evening wore on. Although Brucye was not an avid "animal lover," she was interested in my tales about animals, and in my ambitions to be a veterinarian. I told her about my classes, about Dr. Wilson's hospital, about the Friday night surgery movies.

"That sounds so interesting," she said in her slightly accented voice, and I knew that she was sincere.

"You don't actually have to be in the Pre-Med Club to attend the movies," I said, warming to my topic. "I mean, if you'd like to see them, you could get in with me. Would you like to come with me to the surgery movie on Friday night?"

She did not even hesitate. "Why yes," she said, with her wide, beautiful smile. "I'd like that very much."

Brucye went to the surgery movie with me every Friday night after that. It was not an exciting date, but we both realized that I had a long haul ahead of me to become a veterinarian. Gradually Brucye entered more and more into my plans for the future.

One Saturday, after we had known each other for about three months, we drove out to Thousand Oaks, to a wild animal compound kept by Neil Roosevelt, a distant cousin of the mainline Roosevelt clan. He was a professional animal collector, and spent six months of each year at remote points of the globe, collecting animals. These were sold to zoos and private collectors. Some of the ones kept in Thousand Oaks were used in movie-making.

I had gotten to know Neil Roosevelt, and had visited the compound in Thousand Oaks many times. On the day that I took Brucye out to see it, Neil was there.

"Say, Fred, I've been meaning to call you," he said. "One of my collecting crew has left me, and I'm looking for a man to replace him. We're leaving for East Africa and the Belgian Congo in a month, and plan to be over there for two or three months. What do you say?"

For a moment, I did not know what to say. On the one hand, this offer seemed the chance of a lifetime. On the other hand, there were other chances of a lifetime that might be missed by accepting this one.

I looked at Brucye's face, intently waiting for my answer. "Thanks, Neil, but I can't do it," I said. "I'm embarked on my pre-veterinary studies, and I've got some other things going right now."

Neil looked from me to Brucye, who was smiling again. "Oh well, I see how it is," he said, with a good-humored laugh. "You can't have everything."

Brucye and I were married on July 1, 1956, about a year after we first met. We rented a small apartment in Westwood near the University of California at Los Angeles, and postponed our honeymoon trip for six weeks so I could finish summer school. We planned to drive to Vancouver, British Columbia, Brucye's home town, to get her immigration papers.

Before we left on this jaunt, we decided to invest in a new used car since the old one was not to be trusted on the three-thousand-mile round trip. We settled on a yellow, almost-new Chevrolet convertible, which, according to the salesman, had belonged to Dinah Shore. (Her television show was sponsored by Chevrolet, and she received a new model three times a year, we were told.) What was good enough for Dinah was good enough for us as we set out on our honeymoon trip in a state of unalloyed bliss.

Our drive north was uneventful. We took Highway 99, the main north-south artery through the Pacific states at that time. As we drove up, we noted many roadside animal "attractions" along the way — usually sleazy establishments, offering shows and captive animals for sale.

"On the way back we'll stop," I promised Brucye. "I'd like to get you a raccoon cub. You wouldn't believe how lovable and fun they are."

"That sounds nice," said Brucye, ever the good sport.

It was August, and the sun was hot. Brucye is fair-complexioned, and prone to sunburn. Often we would stop and put the top of the convertible up.

On our return trip, we decided to stop at Crater Lake, in Oregon. The waters in that mountain lake are an incredibly deep shade of blue, and a small island emerges from them, not far from the shore. Even in August there was snow on the ground at that altitude and on the trees on either side of the narrow road. It was cold, and we had the top up on the convertible. I parked under a tree.

"Let's hike down to the lake and get a closer look at the island," I said, eager to stretch my legs.

"Yes, let's," said Brucye. We locked the car and walked over to where the snowy slope descended to the lake below.

Our feet crunched in the snow as we made our way down to that unbelievably blue water. The island had pine trees on it. We stood at the water's edge for awhile, and then hiked back up to the parking lot.

"Oh, Fred!" said Brucye, pointing at our car. The convertible top was caved in under a load of snow, dropped from the tree above!

It was true. We walked around the car, staring in disbelief. As a Southern Californian, I had had little experience with snow. Now I felt incredibly naive.

"Well, we'd better get it off of there, and see what the damage is underneath," I said.

"Right," said Brucye cheerfully, and began shoveling away with her bare hands.

It took us ten or fifteen minutes to clear the broken roof. Snow had gotten inside the car, but the steering wheel and dashboard instruments were undamaged. I was able to fold the top down, and we proceeded down to warmer altitudes.

We stopped at the roadside animal stands in quest of a baby raccoon, but alas, there were none to be had. They had all been born in the spring, and weaned and sold in early summer. Somehow, Brucye did not seem overly disappointed.

We descended California's hot Central Valley in our now permanently open car. When the sun got unbearably hot, Brucye would take the tonneau cover from the roof compartment and crouch under it beside me as I drove. We got some strange looks as we drove along, especially when Brucye would suddenly pop up from beneath her shelter. We laughed at the staring drivers who passed us, enveloped in our own honeymoon bliss.

Just before we reached our apartment, I decided to have one last try for a baby raccoon for my bride. I stopped at a pet shop, and Brucye waited in the car.

No raccoons, but lo! A litter of tiny spotted skunks for sale. Guaranteed descented. I slapped down a crisp twenty-dollar bill, and carried the beady-eyed black and white creature out to the car and presented her to Brucye.

We decided to name our pet "Lotus" — a mild allusion to fragrance, but without any unpleasant connotations. We set up a litter box in the bathroom, and Lotus soon learned to use it. She spent much of her time playing in the bathroom. A favorite game was to stand on her hindlegs beside the tub and slide the shower door back and forth along its metal track. In the wee hours of the night we would lie in bed and listen to the periodic bang of the glass door against its vertical stops.

Another trick of Lotus's, when she was bored, was to excavate her stools from the litter box and play field hockey with them across the tiled floor.

Newly-wed Brucye was a good sport about this initiation into exotic animal husbandry. But to this day, the smell of the pine-scented household cleaners we used to clean Lotus's living quarters has unpleasant associations for both of us.

One day, after we had had Lotus for almost a year, my mother was invited for lunch. These affairs usually went off smoothly, but on this occasion she asked if she could bring her miniature Poodle, "Max," since she would be picking him up at the groomer's on the way.

The doorbell rang. "There she is," said Brucye from the kitchen. "Can you get it?" She was making a cheese soufflé, in my mother's honor.

I opened the door and greeted my parent and her pet, who was fluffed and scented.

"I'm sure he will be no trouble," said my mother, setting Max down on the carpet.

At that moment, Lotus sauntered into the room. Max took one look and charged, yapping excitedly. He had encountered few non-humans in his sheltered life; I doubt that he realized he was a dog.

Lotus took refuge in the bathroom, behind the base of the toilet. Max dove after her, and soon the two of them were whirling around the base of the commode. Lotus weighed about one pound, and her tiny legs carried her easily around and around. Max, being heavier, could not hold such a tight circle, and soon was caroming off the china bowl into the wall and the side of the tub. What fun it was!

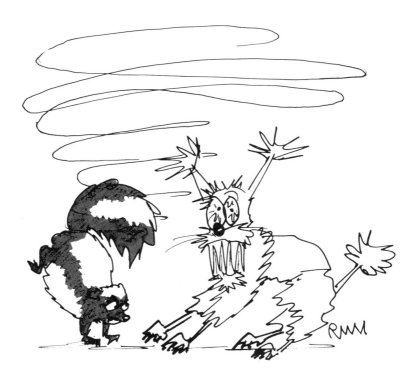

Nothing so entertaining had ever happened to either of the participants, especially Max.

"Fred! Do something!" said my mother from behind me in the doorway.

Before I could intervene, Lotus stopped, stood on her tiny hands, and fanned out her bushy tail. In a movement too rapid to see, she sprayed something into Max's unsuspecting face. Rich, pungent skunk odor filled the room.

"Fred! What's happening?" said Brucye, running from the kitchen. The smell by now had permeated the small apartment. "What's *happening*?"

"Max, my poor Max," said my mother, as her stunned pet stood blinking bewilderedly. She took a towel from the rack and stooping down, wrapped it around him. Gingerly, she picked him up, holding him at arm's length.

"All right, Fred," she said, turning on me, "You're the animal expert. What do we do now?"

"Well, they say that canned tomato juice is the best thing for getting rid of skunk odor," I said cheerfully. "I'll just run down to the corner grocery and get some."

My mother stood, irresolute. Her first instinct was to get out of our richly skunk-scented apartment as fast as possible. And yet, if she put the odor-saturated Max in her car, the smell would surely linger there, and would contaminate her own spotless home.

"All right," she said finally. "But for goodness sake, hurry! And open all the windows before you go."

"I guess we'll have to postpone lunch," said Brucye, glancing wistfully towards the kitchen.

"Thank you, but I don't think I could eat a thing," said my mother. "My appetite is quite gone."

It took numerous washings with tomato juice and then shampoo to bring Max's fragrance intensity down to tolerable levels. Despite repeated cleanings with Pinesol and other agents, the odor of skunk lingered in our apartment for weeks. We made assiduous apologies to all the neighbors, and had Lotus properly descented by Dr. Wilson.

My mother did not visit us for months, and never again with Max!

5 | Veterinarian at Last

Brucye and our two children and I were in the airport at Sacramento.

"When will the new puppy come, Daddy? Is he coming now?" asked three-year-old Lorraine for the hundredth time.

Brucye shifted one-month-old Erik to her other arm and smiled at me.

"He's coming soon," I said. "They just have to unload the baggage, and then they'll bring him to us."

"What's his name?" said Lorraine. "What's his name going to be?"

"We haven't decided yet. We should see him first, don't you think?"

"How big is he, Daddy? Is he just a *tiny* puppy? Is he bigger than kitty?"

"I think he's bigger than kitty," I said wearily. "He's ten weeks old now."

"He's bigger than Erik," said Lorraine wisely. "But not as big as me. I'm three." And she held up three pink fingers.

The object of all this eager questioning was a Bloodhound puppy that Brucye and I had ordered from a breeder in Washington state.

I was finally in my first year of veterinary school, at the University of California at Davis. It had taken me several years to complete my undergraduate studies while both Brucye and I worked part-time to support our family. I had finally completed a Bachelor of Science degree in Animal Husbandry and Animal Physiology. Now I had four more years of veterinary school before earning my Doctor of Veterinary Medicine degree.

Making ends meet while being a student was always touch-and-go, but recently I had hit upon a scheme that seemed made-to-order for us. I had heard that the nearby San Mateo Sheriff's Department paid *one hundred and twenty-five dollars a day* to hire Bloodhounds when searching for missing persons. This, I persuaded Brucye, was an infallible way to bolster our domestic economy.

We got information on various Bloodhound breeders, and began corresponding with some. At that time, Tennessee Ernie Ford's male Bloodhound was seen almost weekly on television. Ford had a trick of grasping a handful of loose skin at the back of the dog's head and pulling it up over its face. The audience always went wild with delight.

"See there," I would say to Brucye, "that's what our hound will look like. We'll have to get a male, of course, since they have more loose skin than the females."

Finally, from photos, we selected a young male from a litter in Washington. Now, today was the appointed day for him to arrive, and it was with great anticipation that we made the short drive from Davis to the Sacramento airport.

"Is that him? Is that him?" Lorraine shrieked as a baggage handler approached with a carrying cage.

It *was* our pup. I lifted him out and gave him a preliminary examination on the spot. He was in excellent health, with questioning brown eyes and a soulful, drooping mouth. He seemed in good spirits, despite his long trip.

"So what is his name?" piped Lorraine as we drove home. "He has to have a name."

"How about 'Hans'?" I said to Brucye.

"So conservative, for a change," murmured my wife.

"Well, if he's going to be a working dog, and go out on assignment, he has to have a serious, short name. We can't have the Sheriff's Department calling 'Here, Meatball!'"

"You're right," Brucye agreed. "'Hans' it shall be."

We were not to learn of the extremely *slow* maturing rate (intellectually) of Bloodhounds until almost a year had passed. To be sure, that blood(y) hound ate a prodigious amount of food, and produced a like volume of droppings, but he retained all of the habits and misdeeds of a puppy. Here he was, all ninety pounds of him, still tearing up the yard and our children's toys, girdling our fruit trees by chewing the bark off all the way around, and destroying clothes hung on the clothesline. At the age of a year, Hans had still not learned to raise his leg to urinate, but squatted like a female.

Once, after Brucye had repeatedly scolded him for dragging clothes from the line, she looked out the window and saw him happily tearing up the clean sheets. Uttering a cry of frustration, she ran out the door and hit the dog over the head with a new broom. The broom-handle broke in half, and Hans, only momentarily cowed, gamboled away.

Greeted with this tale of woe upon my return from school, I moved the clothesline, and decided to take Hans's education in hand. First, etiquette. It was time he learned to raise his leg. Taking him out into the yard in the evening twilight, I alternately lifted his leg and mine, and deposited my own urine on a few low shrubs. Eureka! He actually caught on, and from that day forward, urinated on nearly every non-moving vertical object in his environment.

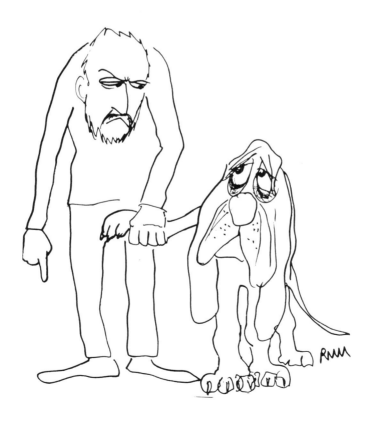

One thing that must be said in Hans's favor — he was good-natured and long-suffering with our children. Once, when he was sleeping peacefully in the kitchen, Erik toddled over and started to climb aboard, using the poor animal's scrotum as a foothold. Hans merely groaned, and shifted his weight.

But as for his Bloodhound's nose, it seemed markedly lacking. He could find his food dish only when he stumbled into it, and then we had to pin his huge ear flaps up over his head with a spring-type clothespin to keep him from eating *them*!

When Hans was sixteen months old, we finally accepted the obvious: we had invested in a *stupid* dog. Had he possessed a brain in that thick but benign skull, we might have persevered. But alas, he was such a dolt.

We could not afford the drain on our slender resources, so we placed an ad for him in the Sacramento paper. At this point, we felt we would be lucky to get back the price we had paid for him.

Two weeks later we received our first inquiry. The caller wanted a male Bloodhound for a breeding program aimed at developing a "superdog" capable of tracking and restraining bears and mountain lions. Twenty minutes later he pulled into our driveway in a pickup truck, with rifle racks spanning the rear window.

I escorted him to the back yard, where he looked Hans over approvingly.

"Does he like cats?" he asked.

"Not particularly," I replied, with a straight face. Actually, Hans and our tabby cat got on quite well, but had a game in which he would chase and tree her in the cherry tree. When he tired of this, he would resume his normal activity: deep sleep and snoring.

"What does he do when he sees cats?" our prospective buyer asked eagerly.

"Oh, he chases them. he's a great chaser. Here, I'll show you."

Brucye materialized on the back step with the cat, primed for action. I chucked the tabby in front of Hans's nose, and she streaked to the nearest tree. As if on cue, Hans charged after her, and since she was out of reach, he threw back his head and howled plaintively. Brucye and I beamed approvingly, and exchanged glances; Hans had never bayed before, except when he heard a firetruck siren. He continued his lament in a series of rising and falling moans, as our visitor listened approvingly.

"I'll take him!" he said, whipping out his checkbook. He paid our price with apparent relish, no doubt thinking he was getting the deal of a lifetime. And perhaps he was, for I later confirmed my suspicions that Bloodhounds mature at a much older age than do Terriers, Retrievers or Spaniels. Hans *may* have grown into a brilliant career of tracking and treeing, and perpetuated his genes in the development of a "superdog." But at the very least, he wasn't still eating our clean laundry!

Our tabby was a stray that had appeared on our doorstep several months previously. Lorraine had named her "Sister Mary." One week after her arrival she gave birth to four healthy kittens. While she was still nursing these, she accepted the attentions of a battle-scarred tomcat and conceived another litter, delivered three weeks after she weaned the first. At this point we renamed Sister Mary "Mother Superior," and I spayed her at the earliest opportunity.

Another cat we adopted was a congenitally spastic cat scheduled to be euthanized at the veterinary school hospital. I brought her home, and we named her "Grace." She was clumsy but lovable, and Lorraine and Erik spent happy hours playing with her. She could, with difficulty, climb stairs, but could never get back down without falling.

After I graduated from veterinary school, we moved to Berkeley, where I had a job with the California Department of Public Health. Brucye and the children and I settled into a house in Kensington, the small hillside suburb adjoining Berkeley.

My position was as "Veterinary Epidemiologist" with the Cancer Research Program. "Epidemiology" is described as "the study of the various relationships of various factors which determine the frequencies and distributions of an infectious process, or a physiological state in a community." Clearly, it is almost easier to *be* an epidemiologist than to describe in one breath the duties of one!

The Program was charged with studying human and animal cancers in the San Francisco Bay area. My job was to maintain contact with all the veterinarians practicing in our study area, and encourage them to submit cases and specimens to us. We maintained a tumor registry where the different cases were categorized and tabulated.

We did not confine our inquiries to domestic animals, and one of the more interesting assignments I had was to autopsy some whales, to check for malignancies.

In 1964 there were still two commercial whaling stations in the continental United States, located next door to each other at Point

Molate, only a few miles from Berkeley. Public outcry against whaling had not yet reached the levels it would later achieve, but one sensed that whaling was a (fortunately) dying industry.

When the opportunity to autopsy whales came along, I leaped at it. Already I was tiring of the pencil-pushing involved in this job, the endless record-keeping of cases submitted by veterinarians out there in real, live practices.

The whaling boats towed their victims back to Point Molate for dissection. I could have fulfilled my job by simply meeting them there, and making my search for tumors. But I had an urge to go along on one of the forays out to sea, and see for myself the whole horrifying drama of whaling.

I talked to the owner of one of the whaling plants, and got permission to go out the following week on the "Del Monte." By coincidence, the skipper, Bud Newton, was the husband of one of the secretaries I knew at the California Veterinary Medical Association.

Armed with an overnight bag, warm clothes, and both movie and still cameras, I joined the rest of the crew in the lonely darkness at Point Molate around 2 a.m. the following Monday. Captain Bud welcomed me aboard the "Del Monte," and introduced the five crew members.

"With luck, we'll be back here by Wednesday night," said Bud, as he started the boat's engines. "We'll be heading due west beyond the Farallon Islands. They're about twenty miles out. We'll keep going another hundred and fifty miles, then range north and south a bit."

"This is an old Navy boat, isn't it?" I said, looking around me and sniffing the smell of rust, tarnished brass, and salt.

"A converted mine-sweeper," said Bud. "She works real well for this job. We can tow two whales on each side, no problem."

The search for whales began at dawn. Contrary to what the ancient mariners thought, whales do not spout water from their blowholes, which are simply modified nostrils closed by a muscular flap. The "spouts" are actually exhaled breath, condensed to mist in the cold Pacific air.

It is possible to determine the type of whale by studying the shape and direction of these exhalations. The killer whale has a single blowhole on the top of its head; the sperm whale's blowhole is located on the left side of the head. The baleen whales, such as the Blue and the Gray, have a pair of blowholes, located symmetrically.

One of the men spotted a spout shortly after 9:30 that morning.

"Looks like a Fin or a Humpback," said Bud, looking through his binoculars. "Of course, it could be a Blue, but they're rare."

There were limits set on each species, set down by the International Whaling Commission, and divided among the nations that maintained whaling industries. The Blue Whales had been decimated in the 1930's, before there were any such controls, and now the limit on them was still low.

"The big whales usually blow several times in a row," said Bud. "Then they'll sound, and stay down ten minutes or more. That's when you get a glimpse at the dorsal fin, or the tail. Humpbacks will lift their tails out when they sound."

The blowing was repeated three or four times, as the creature thoroughly changed the air in its lungs. Then, with a rolling motion, the whale curved its back, and rose partway out of the water. I had a fleeting view of a long, low black fin rising to the summit and descending, as the creature dove.

"It's a Fin Whale, all right," said Bud. "We'll continue on course, and wait for her to blow again."

He turned the wheel over to a crew member, and went down into the bow of the boat, where a cannon held a six-foot harpoon, attached to a coil of wire cable and nylon rope.

"Those harpoons weigh a hundred and sixty pounds," said Bud. "There's a grenade-type mechanism in the tip that explodes on contact. If you get a good hit, they die in about 4 minutes." He paused, and scanned the water. "When you hit a whale in a school, the others stick around and try to help their pal. It's pretty easy, once you find them."

I felt slightly sick as I readied my cameras and we waited for the whale to reappear. They were such peaceful, noble creatures. To kill them and reduce them to pet food, cosmetics and fertilizer seemed unspeakably barbarous.

"There she blows!" shouted one of the crew, as the whale rose nearby. The boat closed in, and at the next rise the cannon thundered. The harpoon shot forward, cut through the water and exploded in the whale's back, embedding the four barbs deep in its body. Blood poured out into the water, eddying around the boat.

"We got her! We got her! It's a Fin, all right."

The huge beast rose slowly to the surface, and floated lifelessly alongside the boat. Its back was dark blue-black, with the low, distinctive fin. The massive head was bowed, and partly submerged in the water.

"Now we pump her full of air, and put a flag on her so we can pick her up on our way home," said Bud, as the men went quickly to work.

"The flag has a radar reflector on the mast so we can find her again even in a fog."

The men made these arrangements quickly, and then we continued on our way, leaving the lifeless body floating with its pennant.

Three more whales were taken in the next thirty-six hours — a Sei, a Humpback, and another Fin-Back. We retraced our course and picked up the victims, which were towed tail first on either side of the boat.

We arrived back at Point Molate around eight o'clock on Wednesday night. The whales were hauled up on the slanting ramp of the plant, and my professional duties began. I had performed necropsies on many species while at veterinary school, but never had been faced with such proportions as these. The Fin-Backs measured about seventy feet long, the Sei and the Humpback around forty-five feet.

The plant's butchers set to work, and I donned coveralls, rubber boots, and a hard hat. The "flensers," men wearing cleats on their boots and wielding hockey-stick-shaped knives, set to work on the first carcass, cutting the attachments between the blubber and the underlying tissue. They needed their special footgear to keep from slipping on the gory surfaces. Forklift trucks and powered chain hoists lifted away huge sections of blubber. Chainsaws cut through bones.

Taking a deep breath, I waded into this massive charnel house. It was mind-boggling. There was the heart, the size of a Volkswagen. Here were the kidneys, larger than bathtubs. This whale was a female, and here were the ovaries, weighing several pounds each. The stomach was huge, and multi-chambered. So far, no sign of tumors.

A proper post-mortem exam includes a thorough search of the body cavities, and at one point I found myself armpit-deep trying to plumb the full depth of the vaginal canal. I tried to extricate my arm, but it was stuck fast in the thick, sticky mucus. Several of the flensers had been watching my efforts with undisguised glee, and finally they rescued me from my predicament!

The butchers swiftly reduced the whale to easily handled portions destined for the pet food, drug, cosmetic and fertilizer industries. It was a disheartening sight.

"Well Fred, you finding anything?" said Bud at one point.

"No tumors so far. I've never seen anything like this," I added, gazing about at this well-organized scene of destruction. "Do you ever eat this stuff?"

"Whale meat? It's great! You can treat it like potroast, or do some other fancy things with it. Maggie marinates strips in buttermilk, and then cooks them like Swiss steak. Here, I'll see that you get some choice cuts."

"Some choice cuts" turned out to be eighty pounds' worth, loaded into my car along with some recipes dictated by Maggie over the phone. I finished my postmortem on the last whale around three o'clock that morning, and headed through the darkness back to Kensington.

I brought the meat into the kitchen, and went to wake Brucye with the good news.

"Fred! You smell like fish!" said my loving wife.

"I'm going in the shower. But wait till you see what's in the kitchen." I ushered her in, and gestured to the eighty pounds of meat.

"Bud says it makes good potroasts," I assured her. I unwrapped a piece, and we looked at it. It was red, with little fat marbling, and no particular odor.

I retired to the shower, and Brucye set to work with every pot and pan she could find to start cooking the fresh meat. Wine, herbs, carrots and potatoes were added to the roasts, which simmered on the stove top and crowded the oven. More meat was cut into strips and set to marinate in the refrigerator.

Finally, after a couple of hours of this unanticipated kitchen activity, Brucye went back to bed.

We were sleeping peacefully when Lorraine and Erik came padding in.

"Mom! Dad! Something smells terrible! What it is?"

"Hmm . . . .?" I dragged myself back to consciousness, aware of a horrible stench. The entire house smelled like a rendering plant. The raw whale meat had had no smell; once cooked, it reeked of rancid fish oil.

Brucye and I ran downstairs, turned off the stove, and opened the windows. I am fond of all seafood, but the smell of this stuff was overwhelming. Bravely, I tried a bite. It was *terrible*! I offered some to our two dogs, and to the cat. They were known to eat *anything*; now they only sniffed and turned away in disgust.

"What shall we do with it?" said Brucye, looking around at all the pots and pans full of cooked meat.

"I'll have to bury it," I said stoically. The hillside where we lived in Kensington was rocky, and digging holes deep enough to discourage raccoons was an effort.

Not one to give up easily, Brucye prepared the whale meat that had been marinating in buttermilk. It was amazingly palatable, as was some whale meat teriyaki she concocted.

However, after this adventure I tactfully declined any more offers of fresh whale meat. I went out on the "Del Monte" a second time, when we brought back a rare Blue Whale weighing more than 200,000 pounds. In all, I necropsied eleven whales at Point Molate. From these, I found two benign growths and two malignant tumors, one of which was a form of leukemia.

I returned to my mundane statistics-gathering job. This was enlivened briefly by my investigation of a multi-cat household that appeared to have a high incidence of cancer among its felines.

In veterinary school, we had heard tall tales about "ailurophiles" — usually women, who gave their entire households over to the care of cats. I assumed that such tales were greatly exaggerated.

I drove the state car up the driveway of the modest rural bungalow, and stopped. The first thing I saw was cats, *everywhere*! On the wooden fence, on the lawn, on the roof, on the front porch. I threaded my way among cats and feeding dishes to the front door.

My knock was answered by a middle-aged woman in blue jeans, carrying a tawny cat.

"Miss Sawyer? I'm Dr. Frye, from the California Cancer Field Research Program in Berkeley." I held out my official credentials.

"I'm so glad you've come," she replied. "Please come in."

I stepped over more feeding dishes into the hallway and stopped, blinking. The air was heavy with the aroma of litter boxes; cat hairs mingled with dust motes in the rays of sunlight penetrating through the open door. A glance to my right showed me a kitchen, with a cat lapping water out of the sink and several companions curled on the counter, the top of the refrigerator, and even on the top of the old-fashioned gas stove.

"We can sit in here," said my hostess, indicating the living room. Stepping over a battery of litter boxes, we entered the room. Every seating surface was already occupied by cats. A gray feline was stretched on the mantlepiece, a tortoiseshell one was curled up on top of the television. Others slept in the sunlight on the threadbare carpet.

"Would you like some tea or coffee?" said Miss Sawyer.

"No, thanks," I said politely, eyeing the pall of cat fur that covered everything. I chose a seat on the sofa that had obviously served as a clawing toy for countless cats. A large black cat shared the cushions with me. Immediately, two creatures came over to rub against my legs and leave hairs behind on my gray flannel trousers.

"I'm so glad you've come," said my hostess again. "I'm sure I know what's killing my cats."

"Oh?" I said, surprised.

"Yes," said Miss Sawyer energetically. "It's well known that smoking causes cancer. And, don't you see" — she paused dramatically — "their cat food has *charcoal* in it! It says so right on the can!" She sat back and began stroking a large gray Manx. "Yes, Matilda," she crooned, "Here's the man who's come to help us."

"Well," I said, somewhat at a loss, "according to the information our office has received, most of your cats died of leukemia or tumors of the lymphoid organs, which is different from lung cancer caused by smoking."

"Cancer is cancer," she said positively. "And charcoal is related to smoke. Isn't that right, Matilda?" The big cat looked at me unwinkingly.

"Well, I'd like to ask you about the medical histories of each of your cats," I continued doggedly. "And about all the humans associated with them, and about the kinds of pesticides and chemicals you use around the house."

"We live alone," said Miss Sawyer. "That is, no other humans. And we've had some terrible losses in the last two or three years, haven't we, Matilda? That's why I telephoned the American Cancer Society."

Slowly, the information emerged. The cats' health troubles had begun three years before, when she was living in San Francisco in an old house that had previously been a cattery. Fleas had been a constant problem, and several cats had been treated for feline infectious anemia, a blood parasite disorder now thought to be transmitted by blood-sucking fleas.

She had moved three times since then, and her second and third homes had also previously been occupied by people with several cats. In the second home, one of Miss Sawyer's pets died of leukemia. As my investigations proceeded, I learned that the occupants of the third home had lost two cats to leukemia. While living there, another of Miss Sawyer's cats had succumbed to the same disease.

At this point, it did appear that we were dealing with a genuine "cluster" of feline leukemia. At that time (1964) feline leukemia was a rarely reported or described disease. Today, the disease complex is recognized quite commonly, and is known to be transmittable from one cat to another. No cases of transmission of leukemia from a cat to a human have been reported.

In the case of Miss Sawyer's household of thirty-four cats, six cases of malignant lymphoma related to feline leukemia, over a period of three and a half years, were confirmed. Five of the six victims were related to one another; the sixth was exposed from the moment it joined the household. The cat food containing charcoal was exonerated.

Two of my veterinary colleagues and I co-authored a report, "A Household Cluster of Feline Malignant Lymphoma," which was published in *Cancer Research* journal. It was the first of several reports on clusters of feline leukemia.

One of the things that relieved the tedium of my pencil-pushing job was the occasional call I got from Steinhart Aquarium, in San Francisco's Golden Gate Park. I was known as a veterinarian with a certain expertise with reptiles, and periodically the senior herpetologist at the aquarium would call me in to treat one of their creatures. These cases were unrelated to cancer research, and I responded to them in my own spare time.

One adventure began with such a call from Karl Switak, the reptile keeper.

"Hi, Fred, This is Karl. We're having a problem with one of the large female alligators in the swamp. Could you come over and have a look?"

Feeling a bit like B'rer Rabbit a'pleading with his tormentors not to throw him into the briar patch, I tried to conceal my excitement at being asked to do what I liked best.

"Sure," I said nonchalantly, "I can drive over tomorrow morning. What seems to be the problem?"

"Well, she's a feisty old gal, and has been getting into a lot of fights with the other 'gators lately. Some of her toes have been chewed up, and I think gangrene may be setting in."

"I see. Okay, Karl, I'll be there around ten o'clock."

At this time, I had had little experience with alligators except for old Pokey and the other smaller crocodilians I'd had in my garage-zoo. In veterinary school we were not taught how to handle alligators, much less how to anesthetize and operate on them. My future patient was surely in the three-hundred-pound class.

Mentally going over the possibilities that evening, I gathered up the equipment and medical supplies I thought I might need. My neighbor, Alan Frankel, often accompanied me on my more interesting missions, and Saturday morning he and I loaded the station wagon and headed across the Bay Bridge to San Francisco.

"Think she'll give you any trouble, Fred?" Alan asked jovially as we drove along.

"No, no. Not with you there to hold her down."

"Me?" said Alan with a laugh from his roly-poly belly. "I'm going to pass you the surgical instruments, remember? I can't do both."

At the aquarium, I donned my rubber boots to wade into the swamp to examine my patient. Two keepers with poles guarded my flanks. A large crowd of Saturday visitors watched these activities with curiosity and excitement.

"Now children," I heard one matron's voice intoning, "you must *never, never* do what that man is doing . . ."

Several of the alligator's toes were indeed gangrenous, and would have to be amputated. "I'd like to take them off right away, so it doesn't spread," I said to Karl. "Where could we move her to do the surgery?"

He thought a moment. "There's a men's washroom down in the basement. It's just been remodeled, and has good lighting."

I agreed. The beast's tooth-studded jaws were bound shut with electrician's tape, and she was hauled onto a litter and carried down to our "operating theater."

Karl Switak was not only the head herpetologist, he was also the largest and strongest man on the aquarium's staff. He sat astride the alligator on the floor, restraining it until I could administer the anesthetic. Another keeper was holding the taped head; two others were in charge of restraining the hindlegs. Alan, too, was crowded into this tiny room, and stood ready to hand me instruments.

The creature never flinched while I cleansed the diseased toes and foot, and applied presurgical antiseptic and sterile drapes. *This*, I thought, *is going to be a piece of cake*.

"Everybody okay?" I asked as I selected a stout hypodermic needle and filled the syringe with anesthetic.

"This old gal isn't going anywhere," said Karl, with confidence born of experience. Indeed, our patient seemed quite lethargic.

I selected a spot near the diseased toes, and inserted the needle between the scales.

The alligator exploded into furious action. Karl was thrown off her back and hit the newly installed toilet, breaking it off at the base and sending the tank through the sheetrock wall. Another of the keepers collided with the sink, sending it partially through the wall. A geyser of cold water shot up from the broken toilet line, and rained down on the scene.

The alligator was thrashing about, the floor was awash, and all five of us humans were trying to get through the narrow door. When I finally made it to the hallway, I looked at my jovial friend Alan. His habitually ruddy face was ashen.

No one was seriously injured in the fracas (or in any other part), but that second or two of utter pandemonium cost the Aquarium over $1,500 in repairs to the bathroom.

Eventually the alligator was restrained sufficiently, transported to another area of the basement, and the surgery was completed successfully.

The next day Brucye read me the account of this escapade in the *San Francisco Chronicle*. Herb Caen, the celebrated columnist, seemed to have a pipeline to every such discomfiting incident, and all of San Francisco was chuckling over the scene in the men's bathroom.

About a year later, when I was in private practice in Berkeley, I operated again on this feisty alligator. This time we had her transported to my hospital, where she was strapped to the table and given anesthesia via a large face mask. She had been the "loser" in another fight, and this time I had to remove an entire rear leg. Now, many years later, she is still alive and well at the Aquarium. She has apparently turned over a new leaf, which is just as well, since she was running out of spare parts!

One of the last interesting assignments I had with the Cancer Research Program was to fly to San Diego to investigate the deaths of several bears living in the same grotto at the San Diego Zoo. This was a treat for me, since the curator of reptiles at this world-famous zoo was an old friend, the late Charles Shaw. As a youngster I had volunteered my services as snake cage cleaner and reptile feeder at the zoo while my parents and sister and I vacationed at nearby Coronado Island.

(Also in those days, I had driven Shaw crazy by trying, when his back was turned, to catch the feral gecko lizards that scurried across the walls and ceilings of the reptile house. Chuck had brought many of these back from expeditions around the world, and most species were thriving and reproducing in their semi-wild state. Geckos shed their tails with ease when threatened with capture, and many bore silent witness to my depradations.)

When I had enlisted in the Navy, I had donated my own animal collection to the San Diego Zoo. It had taken two trips with a loaded car and trailer to empty my garage menagerie.

Now Chuck Shaw welcomed me as a colleague, and when my investigations were over, he presented me with a young reticulated python, one of the first ever bred in captivity. We confined the seven-foot snake in a cloth sack, which I placed in my brown leather briefcase with its "STATE OF CALIFORNIA" embossed in gold on the side. I carried this aboard the plane for the short flight back to San Francisco. Happily for me, this was before the days of pre-flight baggage searches!

The plane was not full, and I chose a spot in the section with three seats abreast. A young sailor in dress blue uniform had the seat by the window. I placed the official briefcase on the empty seat between us, and unzipped it a few inches so my snake would have adequate ventilation.

The stewardess brought us cocktails, and I began to write up my report on the bears. The apparent cause of death was hepatoma, a malignancy of the liver. We traced the cause to a shipment of dried fruit contaminated with *Aspergillum* mold, which produces aflatoxin, a potent liver carcinogen.

About half an hour later, a motion caught my eye. My python, still inside its bag, was pushing its head up through the opening in the briefcase.

I glanced sideways at the sailor and saw that he too was furtively looking at that moving bag. I bent over my papers again, but was aware of him looking from me to the bag and then staring fixedly straight ahead. Silently, he removed his arm from the armrest adjoining the middle seat.

The stewardess passed, and he cleared his throat. *What now?* I thought, with foreboding. Was I going to be denounced here in front of all my fellow passengers? Would the co-pilot be summoned, and stand over me, demanding that I open the briefcase?

"Excuse me, ma'am, but could I have a cup of black coffee?"
He blames the cocktails! I thought, suppressing my delight.

I continued working on my report, the python continued sporadically to emerge from the briefcase, and my seatmate sipped his coffee in stoical silence.

When the plane had taxied to the terminal, I unbuckled my seatbelt, stood up, and took my now-closed official briefcase under my arm. The sailor was beside me as we descended the ramp, but even at this safe moment he never said a word. Obviously he had decided that ignorance of some things was the better part of virtue!

After I had been with the Cancer Research Program for a year, I gave the chief my six-months' notice. I knew that desk work was not for me. The Berkeley Dog & Cat Hospital was for sale, and Jean-Paul Cucuel and I had decided to form a partnership and buy it. He was a Canadian-trained veterinarian who had been working at a local humane society. His particular interest was in caged-bird medicine. Together we could offer the public a wide range of expertise.

In January, 1966, we began our new practice.

6 | The People's Republic of Berkeley

In the ten years that I practiced at the Berkeley Dog & Cat Hospital (1966-76), U.S. involvement in the Vietnam War was at its height, as were student demonstrations. Patty Hearst was a student at UC Berkeley at the time of her famous kidnapping in 1974, and some of her abductors were on our client roster. It was an exciting time to be living in Berkeley, and at times we found ourselves caught up in these events.

In 1969, the increased bombing of North and South Vietnam set off a series of violent demonstrations in Berkeley. For a few incredible days, the business district of the town resembled an armed camp. The streets were patrolled by hastily mobilized, youthful National Guardsmen with bayonet-fixed rifles, blue-clad state policemen (called the "blue meanies" by the street people), and policemen in gas masks and flak jackets. Machine gun-equipped jeeps and camouflage vehicles cruised the streets.

Berkeley residents responded with a wide spectrum of emotions, not always determined by age. Many older citizens expressed bewilderment and disgust at the civil disobedience shown by some younger demonstrators, others vociferously supported them. Many young people tried to prevent the wanton destruction of public and private property; others delighted in hurling garbage, paint, dung and bricks at the representatives of law and order.

Berkeley Dog & Cat Hospital was located near the center of the turmoil. More than once, tear gas and other chemical agents were drawn into our central ventilation system. Preoccupied with a patient, I would suddenly become aware of the acrid odor and a smarting of the eyes, as tears formed uncontrollably. When this happened, we would turn on the air conditioning, which would quickly dilute and dissipate the chemical.

Several dogs were brought to us after having been sprayed directly with the "crowd control" agents. The creatures were frantic, their eyes streaming and their mouths drooling uncontrollably. We would flush their eyes out and calm them, and send them back into the embattled streets.

A cat was brought to us after ingesting a yellow phosphorous fuse from a tear gas canister. It subsequently died of the poison.

During those turbulent days, our clients had to pass through a gauntlet of National Guard and police checkpoints to reach our hospital by car. I will always be grateful to those loyal people who were willing to do this instead of going to a veterinary hospital in a less troubled area.

One day a roving gang of gratuitous "protestors" laid siege to a small Chinese laundry next door to our modern hospital building. Armed with paving stones, bricks and a baseball bat, they "trashed" the premises and the modest car of the elderly proprietor.

Summoned from the back by our receptionist, Denny Hoeft and our resident, Jay Stone, and I rushed out front in our white uniforms. The gang, tiring of their easy "victory" next door, were eyeing our large expanse of plate glass windows. Jay is another six-footer, and he and Denny and I lined up with our backs to the window, a formidable white phalanx. The motley crew hesitated and then drifted on down the street, in search of easier prey.

One night I had an excited call from Johnny.

"Dr. Frrrye, there's been an explosion somewhere nearby. I'm afraid some of our windows are brroken! Ye'd best come doon."

I arrived to find several plate glass windows on the east side of the building shattered. While Johnny swept up the glass, I went home for some sheets of plywood. Johnny and I stacked these against the opening, and then calmed the agitated animals. Contemplating the scene, I could not help thinking, "No one told me that private practice would be like this!"

The next morning we called the glass company, which was doing a brisk business. The explosion had been a bomb set off in the anti-war Vietnam Day Committee Headquarters, around the corner from us. That building was completely destroyed.

Shortly after this, we had special heavy wooden shutters built to completely cover the plate glass windows on the front of the building. Our insurance company recommended this move. At the first hint of trouble, we could put the shutters up.

In our practice, the Vietnam War also had an effect on our own war on fleas. At that time, the most effective flea control products were made by a little-known subsidiary of the Dow Chemical Company. In anti-war circles, Dow was synonymous with napalm, the jelly-like, hellish fiery sustance rained down on the population in Southeast Asia. Some of our clients discovered that Dow was indeed the parent company of the manufacturer of the flea products, and so refused to buy or use any of these.

I was certainly not a supporter of the war, but since I had a duty to my patients, I was frustrated at not being able to prescribe the insecticides I knew would help them the most. It was a curious intersecting of politics and veterinary medicine.

We finally returned most of these flea products to the distributor, along with a frank explanation of the problem.

Later, I asked some local grocers if their sales of Saran Wrap, another Dow product, had declined. They had not. Apparently plastic wrap is indispensable, even to zealots. Flea control ranks lower on their list of priorities!

Another paradox of the anti-war movement in Berkeley concerned the matter of dress. Even the most ardent pacifists made their stand arrayed in army surplus clothing. Only a few times did the irony seem deliberate. One day as I passed a demonstration, I saw two young men in GI field jackets. On the back of one was stenciled "PAX;" on the other, "NIHIL." The irony had a disturbing poignancy.

About the time of the North Vietnamese and Viet Cong Tet offensive, Brucye and I were in a shopping mall, riding an escalator. As we ascended, I glanced down at a bit of graffiti that some sage had recently scrawled. Perhaps better than anything else, it summed up the tenor of the times. It read (after some genteel editing): "BOMBING FOR PEACE IS LIKE FORNICATING FOR CHASTITY."

Such microcosmic vignettes exemplify what Berkeley was then, is now, and probably shall forever be.

On February 4, 1974, Patty Hearst, heiress daughter of the newspaper publishing magnate, was kidnapped in Berkeley. The abductors were part of a small band who called themselves the Symbionese Liberation Army. As the identity of these urban guerillas was made known through the press, I was amazed to recognize the names of two former clients of mine.

William and Emily Harris, credited by the press with being leaders of the movement, had been coming to me for eight years with a series of cats. I had seen the small, blond Emily more often than I had seen Bill. I considered her an intelligent, conscientious pet-owner.

Others of the band, Patricia ("Mizmoon") Soltysik, Camilla Hall, and Nancy Ling Perry had had pets treated by my colleagues.

We watched the drama unfold in the press as Patty Hearst re-emerged as "Tania," a seeming convert to the band and an accomplice in a successful bank robbery in San Francisco that April. The impassive-faced Tania was photographed by bank cameras as she held an automatic weapon.

On the Saturday following these events, Denny Hoeft and I finished at the hospital and stepped out into the parking lot. Two men in gray suits and wearing identical aviator-style sunglasses stood before us displaying FBI credentials. They asked if they could come in and talk with us.

Somehow the FBI had picked up a lead that several members of the SLA had been our clients, and they wanted to search our records. As it turned out, all of the members of the gang had moved from the addresses listed in our records some time before.

Later, FBI agents searched our records a second time, hoping to find distinctive pet names or medical histories that veterinarians in other parts of the country could be alerted to watch for. The gang had gone underground, and presumably was on the run. Possibly they still had their pets in tow. As it turned out, nothing came of this lead.

One month later, in May, we watched with horror as television brought us the spectacle of the SLA's last stand in the house in Los Angeles. TV screens across the country lit up as sheets of flame engulfed the house, burning it to the ground before our eyes. All six members of the band who were in the house perished, holding out to the last in the crawl space beneath the floor.

Later, it was revealed that Patty Hearst and the Harrises were not with the others at the time of the shoot-out. It was many, many months later that they were apprehended, once more in the Bay Area.

Drugs were another dark side of the scene in Berkeley and San Francisco. Several times we were brought animals that had been given marijuana, LSD, mescaline, peyote, phencyclidine ("angel dust"), methamphetamine, or heroin. Since our first duty was to the patient, we treated the animals without reporting the incident to the authorities. Had we done so, we would have seen no more of these abused creatures who needed care.

One of these was an accidental case of marijuana ingestion. A youth and two young girls brought in a comatose Shepherd puppy. According to the history card, the pup had "experienced a sudden loss of activity."

I examined the animal as the trio stood by uneasily. The dog was breathing very slowly, the pulse was low, and the rectal temperature was slightly lower than normal.

"Could he have gotten into any prescription drugs?" I asked. The three young people shook their heads.

As soon as I opened the puppy's mouth, I spotted some plant material, and smelled the distinctive peppery odor of *Cannabis sativa* (marijuana).

"Uh huh, it looks as if your puppy has been eating something other than puppy chow."

One of the girls giggled, the other began to cry. The youth grinned broadly.

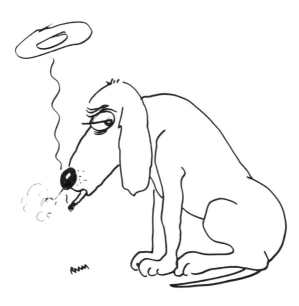

"Oh Dr. Frye," sobbed the girl, "we didn't know it would affect Geezer so horribly. We're so sorry. Please don't tell on us."

I assured them that their secret would remain within that room, but asked for details so I could treat the stupefied animal.

They had apparently bought some unrefined marijuana, still containing stems and seeds. They had picked out the usable leafy parts, and disposed of the chaff in a bag in the garbage can. The puppy had found this beneath the sink, and had eaten the entire bagful, much to their amusement.

I flushed the potted puppy from one end to the other, and administered respiratory stimulants. He soon was fully recovered, with an enormous appetite. It would seem that dogs as well as humans experience the post-marijuana "munchies!"

We had several clients whom we suspected of being members of "the underground economy" — the drug-dealing culture that flourished in that time and place.

Frank was a streetwise former New Yorker. He first appeared in our hospital one day with his spayed German Shepherd bitch, Angel.

"Have you been here long?" I asked as I examined the dog.

"Awhile," he replied. "Stopped in Chicago awhile before we hit this scene. Drove out in the van. M'wife, our kid, m'wife's sister."

I finished treating the dog. "Whaddo I owe yuh?" Frank said, removing a heavy roll of currency from his pocket.

"You can pay at the receptionist's desk," I said, trying not to stare.

"Right." He shoved the wad back in his pocket, and snapped his fingers at the dog. "Angel!" The dog moved towards the door.

Frank and Angel came in several times, and he always paid in cash from a large roll. Hattie would watch silently as he peeled the bills off, reluctant to summon up her usual flow of cheerful small talk.

A few months after I had left the practice to pursue graduate studies at the University of California at Davis, I read in the paper of a drug-related multiple murder in Berkeley. The victims, who were stabbed to death, were Frank, identified as a major drug dealer, his wife, her sister, and the dog, Angel.

Unfortunately, in the early 1970's such events were not rare.

In Berkeley, the diversity of the population was reflected in the names given to pets. At one end of the spectrum, we saw many drug-scene-inspired names: "Hash," "Roach," "Sniff," "Munchie," "Smack," "Stash," and even "Zig Zag," named for the popular cigarette paper in which marijuana joints are frequently rolled.

At the other end of the spectrum, from the academic community, we saw pets with classical, literary, or music-inspired names. "Othello" and "Desdemona" were a pair of Terriers, one black, one white. Two cats belonging to a physicist were named "Quark" and "Quasar." "Ebb" and "Flo" were two Poodles belonging to a professor of hydrology. A professor of naval science called his two cats "Flotsam" and "Jetsam."

The chief of urology at a nearby hospital named his two Burmese cats "Phyllis" and "Phallus." "Null" and "Void" were a pair of nondescript alley cats owned by two attorneys. A meteorologist friend of mine called his two Dachshunds "Fair" and "Warmer." Another attorney called his two cats "Cease" and "Desist." Our dentist's two cats were "Flossie" and "Carie." A gynecologist client named her neutered tomcat "Venus Envy."

Then there was a couple named Beame, who called their pair of Yorkshire Terriers "High" and "Low." They also had a big, very sleek cat named "Jim." Similarly, we saw "Snow" White, "Small" Frey, and "Genghis" Cohen, a great gray tomcat who was the scourge of his neighborhood.

I saw more than one boa constrictor named "Julius Squeezer," and not a few "Monty" Pythons. One creative owner, who carried her boa around her shoulders, called him "Feather."

"Dropshot" was a full-grown African cheetah, whose owner was a professional tennis player. He transported the big cat to and from the hospital in the front of his open convertible, where it always caused quite a stir.

I was not above playing the name game. When I was studying the metabolism of several species of bats, I kept two examples in cages in my study, "Batman," and "Robin." We also had a desert tortoise named "Uriah;" he looked like a heap. Our scroungy mongrel dog was named "Shibui" — Japanese for "understated elegance."

A new client once appeared with a cat whose name, according to the record card, was "Alles." Hearing the woman's heavy accent, I asked if the receptionist had misunderstood the animal's name.

"Nein, nein, Herr Doktor," the portly matron replied. "Zis kitty is goingk to be ze last vun." Smiling benignly, she veritably gushed, "Ja, das ist Alles!"

I wonder how many others she caught with that awful but wonderful pun!

There were two lively Siamese cats, "Pande " and "Monium." And two Southeast Asian slow lorises, "Boris" and "Doris." And a pair of Pakistani hedgehogs named "Paki" and "Stan."

In the bird world, we had a toucan with a prominent beak, named "Cyrano." There was a parrot named "Esther;" with her well-preened plumage, she was "Pollyesther!" Another small parrot was called "Chicken George," after the character in *Roots*.

I think my favorite name over the years was that of a parrot who had learned to mimic the sound of the household vacuum cleaner. This beady-eyed fowl went by the name of "Hoover Upright!"

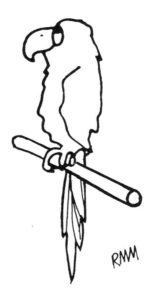

7 | Expedition to the Indus

Dr. Earl Herald was looking at me speculatively, as I sat across from him in his office at Steinhart Aquarium. I had dropped by for my weekly "house call" to the reptiles, amphibians, and aquatic mammals at the Aquarium. But instead of wrestling with alligators in the swamp, I was seated in the office of the chief. Dr. Earl Herald was a marine biologist with an international reputation, and well-known to San Francisco television viewers for his weekly science programs.

Earl leaned back in his chair.

"Say, Fred, I know you've had a lot of experience treating animals," he said conversationally. "Have you ever taken any human medicine courses?"

"Only tropical medicine," I said, surprised. "I took a few courses at the University of California."

"You did!" Earl's eyes brightened; he seemed inordinately pleased with this information. He gazed into space for a few moments.

"You had much experience with dolphins?" he continued, in an apparent change of subject.

"Not a lot. I've treated a few of the porpoises here. That's about it. In fact, the only marine mammals I've treated are the harbor seals here, 'Butterball,' your manatee, and that baby South American manatee that died the day after it arrived."

"Well — yes," said Earl absent-mindedly. "But I'm not talking about *salt-water* dolphins. Have you ever heard of the fresh-water, platanistid dolphins that inhabit the rivers of India and Pakistan?"

"I can't say that I have."

"They're called 'blind' dolphins," said Earl, his eyes sparkling with interest. "The water they live in is so silt-laden that they apparently get around by means of sonar. Or so it is believed. None have ever been brought to the Western Hemisphere for study."

He reached for a sheaf of papers on his desk. "The point is, I now have a grant. A grant to go to Pakistan and study these creatures. And, if I'm lucky, to bring one or two back here with me."

I sat forward eagerly in my chair. This was the stuff that a zoologist's dreams were made of!

"I need someone who can help with the studies, and help get any live specimens back here in good health."

I nodded, in a daze.

"The thing is," said Earl, "I also need someone who can serve as the party's physician. We're going to be in a fairly remote area, and anything could happen." He looked at me intently. "Do you think you could handle that? We'll be out of the country, so there would be no problem over practicing medicine on humans without a license."

I sat silent for a moment. Nearly fifteen years before, I had turned down Neil Roosevelt's invitation to join him in trekking around the world collecting animals. Then, I was just getting to know Brucye, just getting started in my pre-veterinary studies. Now, I had been in practice for more than two years, and had taken only one week of vacation in that time. Opportunity, it seemed, was defying the proverb and knocking a second time.

"I'll have to talk to my wife and my colleagues at the hospital," I said, trying to suppress my excitement. "When are you going?"

"It looks like next fall," said Earl. "It will probably take four to six weeks, depending on how hard it is to locate and capture the creatures. I'm in touch with an Anglo-Pakistani fellow, Cedric Watson*, in Karachi. His business is collecting animals for zoos. He has organized this kind of expedition before. He'll make all the arrangements on that end."

I sat spellbound as Earl filled in the details. The grant money had originated from the U.S. Navy's Bureau of Undersea Warfare. It was channeled through the Smithsonian Institution to the California Academy of Sciences, the parent organization of the Steinhart Aquarium. (Although this arrangement appears convoluted, covert, and even sinister, it is not an unusual one, when a study can benefit several unconnected agencies.)

"The Navy apparently wants to study the potential bio-sonar capabilities of these dolphins," said Earl.

---

*Name has been changed to protect his identity in Pakistan.

I thought back fleetingly to my eight years of active and reserve duty in the Navy. Imagine fulfilling one's military obligation studying dolphins! Obviously, I had been born too soon.

There were added embellishments to the expedition. A while back, His Imperial Highness, Crown Prince Akahito of Japan had visited the Steinhart Aquarium. He was a respected zoologist, specializing in ichthyology (the study of fishes), like Earl. He had extended an invitation to Earl to stop in Tokyo and visit his country's several public aquaria, which were renowned for their innovative displays and wide variety of species.

Earl had also arranged a stop in the Philippines, where the United Nations Food and Agriculture Organization had commissioned him to inspect some aquaculture and mariculture projects.

In Thailand, another official stop would revolve around inspecting a famous collection of preserved fish, on behalf of the Vanderbilt Foundation, which had funded the original project.

As I sat listening to this itinerary of zoological delights, I could hardly contain my excitement. I could see the pages of the National Geographic coming to life before my eyes. I *had* to go!

There were to be two other members of the party, Bob Brownell, a graduate student in cetology (the study of whales, porpoises and dolphins), and Elkan Morris, an amateur herpetologist from Alaska, who was planning to film the expedition for a possible TV program.

"So you see, Fred, we can't afford both a veterinarian and a physician," said Earl. "I don't know any MDs who could treat a porpoise," he smiled, "so the choice comes down to you. I'd feel safe in your hands, and I know Bob and Elkan would agree."

That night Brucye and I sat up talking half the night. The next day I talked to my partner, Jean-Paul Cucuel. It was decided. I was to join the expedition to the Indus River, in West Pakistan.

This was 1968. An earlier plan to study the dolphins in the Ganges River in northern India had been changed after the political climate in that area became too unsettled. The government of West Pakistan, under the presidency of General Mohammad Ayub Khan, invited us to come to their country and study the dolphins in the Indus River, in the Baluchistan region. After making our official stops in Japan, the Philippines and Thailand, we would fly to Karachi, in West Pakistan. The West Pakistani Navy had sanctioned our expedition to some militarily sensitive areas on the Indus river. As we understood it at the time, our own Department of State tacitly, if not expressly, supported our plans.

I took my role as prospective physician seriously. What eventualities should I prepare for if we were to be camped out in a remote spot?

I bought four large fishing tackle boxes, and proceded to stock them. Since one of my interests in practice was conducting new drug trials for several pharmaceutical companies, I had many contacts in that industry. When told of the upcoming expedition, many companies generously donated supplies.

Starting at the basic level, I laid in supplies of antidiarrheal and antinausea medication, cough and headache remedies, antihistamines, and burn ointments. More soberly, I packed in splints, plaster of Paris cast materials, and local and general anesthetics. I packed in three sterile surgical instrument packs, a dozen pairs of sterile surgical gloves, and several sterile surgical gowns, masks, caps, and towels and drapes. I signed out a modest supply of Demerol, a powerful narcotic painkiller, from our safely guarded store.

From our veterinary hospital's supplies I borrowed surgical tubing and syringes, intravenous fluids, infusion sets, needles and suture materials, and miscellaneous ophthalmologic and dental gear. I planned to bring back all the surgical and diagnostic instruments, but to donate any unused drugs and bandage materials to the human hospital at Karachi, just before we returned.

When my portable "field hospital" was packed in the four tackle boxes and lined up next to my other luggage, I looked like a jetsetting sportsfisherman, off on an extended jaunt. (This year the rivers of Pakistan, maybe next year, the lochs of Scotland . . .)

To facilitate getting all these drugs through customs, I typed inventories to accompany each box, and gave a copy of this manifest to the U.S. customs superintendent at San Francisco International Airport. Once through customs, each box was sealed and padlocked before being loaded on the plane.

Fortunately, no one ever questioned the pharmacy bottles labeled "Medicinal Spirits" that were tucked behind the gauze bandage materials. These contained bonded bourbon and Scotch whiskey, and none was left over to donate to the hospital in Karachi!

Earl and Elkan Morris and I left San Francisco in October, 1968. Bob Brownell, the cetology student, was to meet us in Tokyo. He had been studying in the Soviet Union. Elkan was to be in charge of shooting movie footage; I was the official "still" photographer.

We settled back in our seats and sipped our drinks.

"How do you feel about eating the native food, Fred?" said Elkan.

"I'm pretty much omnivorous," I replied confidently.

"How about you, Earl?" said Elkan.

"Well, I'm making no promises," said our chief, cautiously. "You've brought along plenty of antidiarrheals, Fred?"

"Yes, sir. Here's hoping we won't need them."

Earl shook his head and raised his glass.

"How about a pact, Fred," continued Elkan. "How about we make a deal right now that we'll eat anything that's set before us, no matter what?" Elkan was from Alaska, and no doubt had eaten some unorthodox things in his time.

I was game. "It's a deal. I'm ready for anything." We shook hands solemnly, then broke into spontaneous laughter. Four weeks of adventure lay before us — exotic places and people and animals, and a scientific challenge. We had planned this trip for nearly a year, and now we were on our way!

"Say," said Elkan seriously, "before we get to Thailand, I think we ought to practice singing their national anthem. Some friends of mine who were over there taught it to me. It dates from the time Thailand was still the Kingdom of Siam."

"Oh?" said Earl, surprised.

"Yes. The words are *Ah wah tah gu Siam,* and they're sung to the same tune as *My country 'tis of thee.*"

"Really?" said Earl. "Remarkable. I thought oriental music--"

"Never mind," said Elkan hurriedly. "Let's just try it out, in case we're ever called upon to join in the singing."

"Okay," Earl said with a shrug, and he and I dutifully sang, "Ah, what a goose I am," to the great entertainment of some of the nearby passengers.

Comprehension dawned slowly on us, and Elkan beamed in approval. "You guys are great!" he said. "Now we're ready for anything!"

There was a fuel stop in Honolulu, and we went to stretch our legs in the terminal. Tacked to the Pan Am message board was a note for Earl. Dr. Herald was requested to phone the following number. He excused himself to the nearest phone booth, and Elkan and I looked at postcards.

Ten minutes later, Earl returned, his face red, his blue eyes sparkling angrily.

"I got some third-hand message, allegedly from the State Department. We are requested to stay here, and not go on to Pakistan!"

"What?" I shouted, as Elkan stared, dumbfounded. "You've got to be kidding!"

"No explanation, no clarifications!" fumed Earl. "I say, forget it! Our government gave its blessing to this project. The Pakistani government has invited us. And we have important commitments along the way. We'll keep going, and see what happens."

Elkan and I agreed heartily. We boarded the plane, and headed for Tokyo.

At Haneda Airport, south of Tokyo, we were again greeted by a note requesting Earl to call the following number. Elkan and I waited at the luggage claim.

"What do you suppose the story is this time?" I said as we waited for our bags to appear. "I don't understand it, after all our preparations."

"Maybe it's the CIA," said Elkan, and we both laughed.

Earl returned with the same message as in Hawaii, and still no explanation. "But they haven't actively prevented us from coming this far," he said cheerfully. "I say, let's keep going until they stop us."

I spotted my brown Air Force-style canvas suitcase descending on the conveyor belt. Funny, it seemed to have a dark stain on the side, that had not been there before. As I seized it, I smelled a strong, brewery-like smell.

It was sake! Some fellow-traveler had apparently packed a bottle of the rice wine in his luggage, and this had leaked onto my bag. (Talk about carrying coals to Newcastle: who would *bring* sake into Japan?)

I did not open my bag there, for as guests of the Imperial House, we were met by a member of the Prince's staff, and whisked through customs.

At the hotel, I unzipped my suitcase with trepidation. I had packed one good suit for state occasions; the rest were casual work clothes. I lifted the canvas flap, and there was my suit, neatly folded, soaked, and reeking.

"Look at this!" I groaned to Elkan, who had the adjoining suite. "We're supposed to be at the Crown Prince's palace in two hours! How am I going to get this thing presentable?"

"Maybe you should hustle out and buy a new one."

"Are you kidding? There aren't too many six-foot three-inch people around here. There wouldn't be anything my size."

"Call the hotel's valet service, and see if they can help."

A few moments later, a small Japanese man in the hotel's uniform was at the door.

"Can you do something about this?" I said in desperation, displaying the beleagured suit. "I need it by seven o'clock. We're going to visit His Imperial Highness Crown Prince Akahito, and Princess Michiko."

The man's eye's widened. "His Imperial Highness? Yes, sir, very good, sir. I will see. I will be back in one-half hour." And bowing slightly, he departed with the offending garments.

The man did a noble job, and managed to steam out most of the sake. To be sure, there was more than a hint of mint swirling about my person as we set out for the royal residence.

We were chauffeured to the Prince's home in a black Cedric sedan. Later, we learned that only the cars of high-ranking government officials are black. (As we thought about it, we realized that we had never seen any black Datsuns or Toyotas at home.)

The Prince's home was the epitome of elegance and simplicity. We left our shoes at the door as we entered. (None of us was small, but I imagine that my size thirteen shoes provided the most cause for merriment among the interested servants!)

Prince Akahito greeted us in his excellent English. He was dressed in a Western-style suit, but his wife, Princess Michiko, wore a beautiful silk kimono. She spoke little English, but smiled graciously. We knelt on tatami mats, to partake of the traditional tea ceremony.

The tea was accompanied by sweets — the first challenge to Elkan's and my gastronomical pact, and not a formidable one. They were clear, gelatinous squares, some green, some yellow, some red, and made from agar. We downed several with the tea, as we talked about marine mammals and fish.

The Crown Prince's area of special interest is in goby fish, a family of elongated, spiny-finned fishes found in nearly all the oceans and in some brackish water not far from the sea. (The California "mudfish" — *Gillichthys mirabilis* — is a goby.)

The Crown Prince's father, Emperor Hirohito, is also a renowned zoologist and marine biologist. He has written several books on his area of particular interest, a family of marine gastropod mollusks called nudibranchs. Another son, brother of the Crown Prince, is also a highly respected naturalist.

The Crown Prince had lined up many zoological treats for us. One morning, his personal chamberlain, a stately white-haired man, arrived at our hotel at 4 a.m. to take us on a tour of Tokyo's central fish market.

As at Les Halles in Paris and Covent Garden in London, the action at this huge market goes on well before dawn, so that storekeepers can procure their produce before the shoppers are out.

It was raining as the black car disembarked us and our guide at the huge collection of sheds that cover more than a square mile of floor space. Inside, dim light bulbs strung from the ceiling lit an incredible scene.

Acres upon acres stretched in every direction, teeming with sea life of every sort. There were tanks of live turtles, snakes and eels. Crabs and prawns scuttled about in tubs of brine. Other tanks held scurrying limpets and live top shells. Displayed on ice-packed trays were freshly caught octopus, dolphin and whale meat. Other counters displayed dried fish and seaweeds, and other mysterious parchment-like objects.

In and among these delicacies thronged the buyers, speaking in the rising and falling tones of their native language. The smell of brine, fish and seaweed was pungent and exhilarating in this pre-dawn, chilly atmosphere.

After we had seen all the sights in the world's largest fish emporium, the chamberlain proposed that we walk to the nearby docks and observe the ritual of fugu dissection.

Fugu is the generic name applied to several species of very poison-ous puffer fish. A lethal toxin, tetrodotoxin, is contained in the mucoid slime covering their bodies and in some of the internal organs, especially the liver and ovaries. If these are excised immediately, before the poison can leach to the surrounding flesh, the meat is edible, and a great delicacy to fugu enthusiasts. We learned that there was an arcane mystique to eating fugu.

"Sounds like playing Russian Roulette with chopsticks," said Bob as we strolled along the dock. I agreed, thinking uncomfortably of Elkan's and my pact to eat anything offered.

(Later, we discovered that the allure of the fugu went far beyond the piquancy of risking death with every bite.)

"These are fugu fins," said the chamberlain, pointing to spiny fins nailed all over the wall of a wooden shed. "When they are dry, fugu-lovers will put them in sake. They soak a long time, then people drink. There is not very much poison in the fins."

Elkan and I exchanged glances. Surely we would not be offered anything lethal?

Our guide ushered us aboard a small fishing boat moored to the dock. Here, licensed fugu dissectors were swiftly and meticulously (one hoped!) plying their trade.

"Fugu dissectors study for three years," said the chamberlain. "They study anatomy and physiology of all the fugu." He smiled a broad, even-toothed smile.

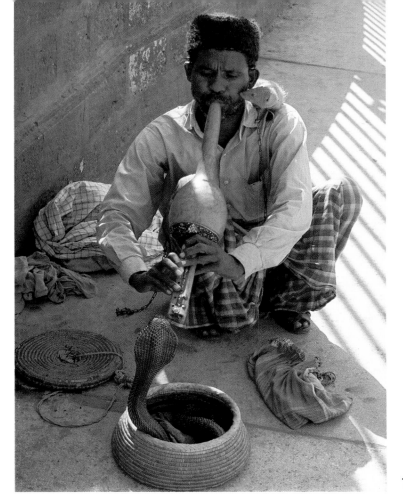

1

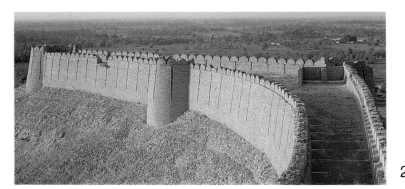

2

Figure 1. A typical street scene -- A flute-playing snake charmer is ready to entertain with a mock battle between his faithful mongoose and the cobra.

Figure 2. The northwest-facing wing of the magnificent Moghul fort, Kot Digi.

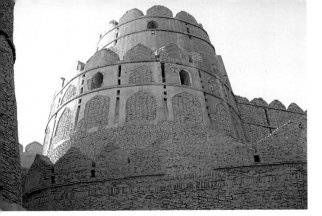

3

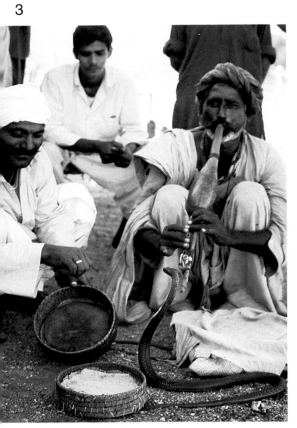

5

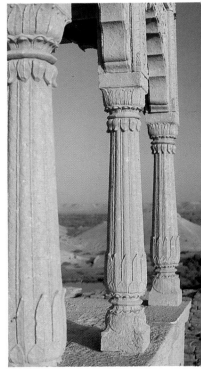

4

Figure 3. A crenelated and parapet-topped tower that demonstrates the exquisite mortar-free masonry construction.

Figure 4. Detail of carved sandstone construction. In the background can be seen numerous raised stupas, believed to be ancient burial sites.

Figure 5. A Joghi demonstrates his prowess with a freshly caught cobra in our camp on the Indus River.

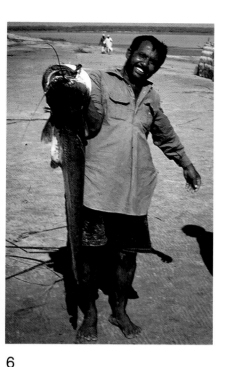

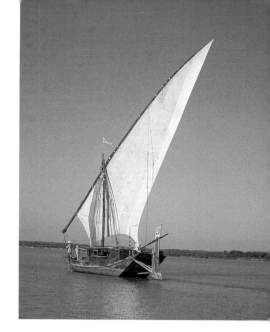

7

6

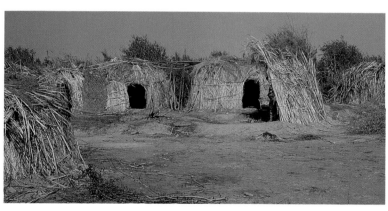

8

Figure 6. Natha, a Sindi fisherman who worked for us, proudly shows off his prize catfish that he caught in a bow net.

Figure 7. One of the shallow draft boats which brought us to camp. These boats are often towed along the banks by a crewman walking on the shore.

Figure 8. Shown here is disposable housing unchanged in design for thousands of years. When the fisher people move, the houses are usually burned and new dwellings are built on another site. A very practical way of preventing vermin and filth-borne diseases.

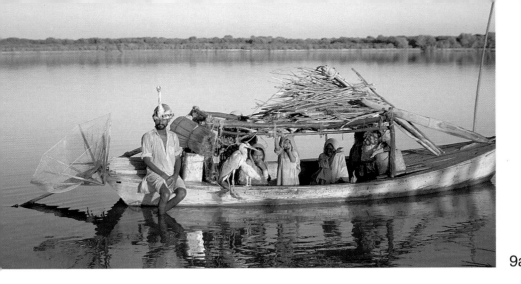

9a

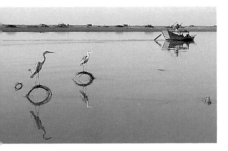

9b

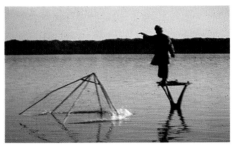

9c

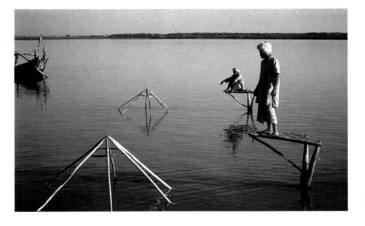

9d

Figure 9a-d. The "Heron People" of the lower Indus River live most of their lives in these tiny boats. They employ wild-caught herons to catch fish. They obtain these herons by submerging themselves in shallow water wearing decoys on top of their heads (as pictured in figure 9a) and then grabbing a heron by its legs. Figure 9b shows a pair of captive herons that are tethered to woven reed bows. These fascinating people also use the bow net (Figures c & d) to catch fish, small turtles, freshwater shrimp, etc.

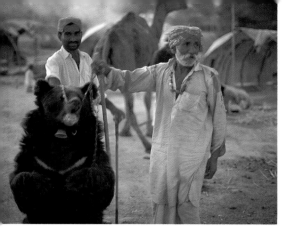

10

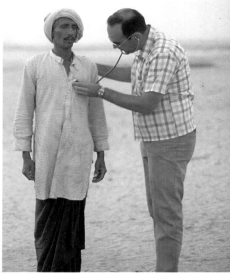

11

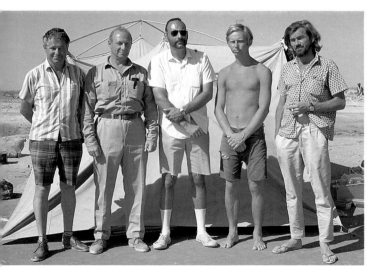

12

Figure 10. A trained bear is being induced by a Joghi to perform by having a lanyard that passes through his upper lip pulled. The camel remains the major beast of burden.

Figure 11. Sick-call at our base camp. There is never a shortage of patients.

Figure 12. From left to right Earl Herald, Elkan Morris, the author, Bob Brownell, and Jerry Anderson.

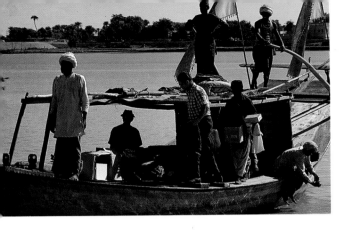

13

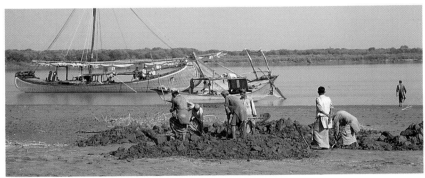

14

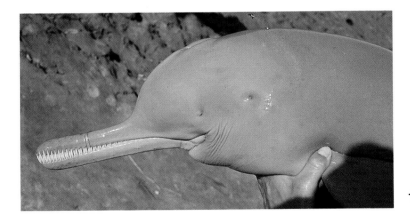

15

Figure 13. Readying our vessel for our first foray to capture blind platinistid dolphins.

Figure 14. Some of our crew digging a holding pool on the banks of the Indus River.

Figure 15. Close-up detail of a blind platinistid dolphin. The native word is buhlaan; in Urdu they are called Susu. Note the many long and very sharp teeth with which these small cetaceans catch their prey. The skin-covered eye is seen immediately above the corner of the dolphin's mouth; the larger depression is the left ear.

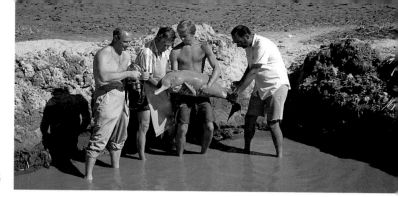

16

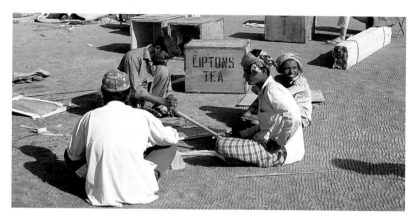

17

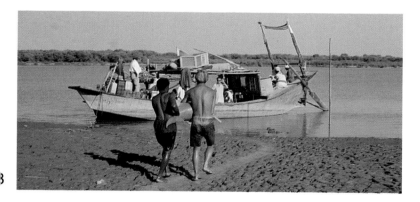

Figure 16. We monitored and treated our dolphins daily. The center of the pond was deeper than the edges so that our precious captives could swim comfortably. From left to right: Elkan Morris, Earl Herald, Bob Brownell, and the author.

Figure 17. Here tea boxes are being disassembled and reassembled into shipping crates that were used for our three dolphins' 14,000 mile trip to San Francisco.

Figure 18. Bob Brownell and Natha carry one of the dolphins to our boat on the day of departure.

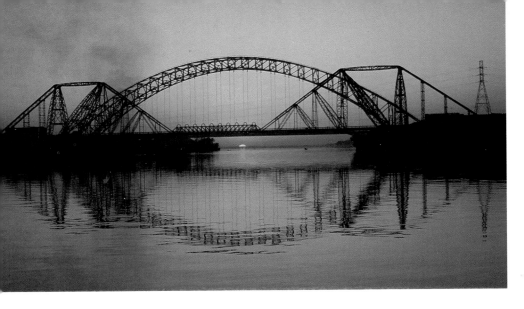

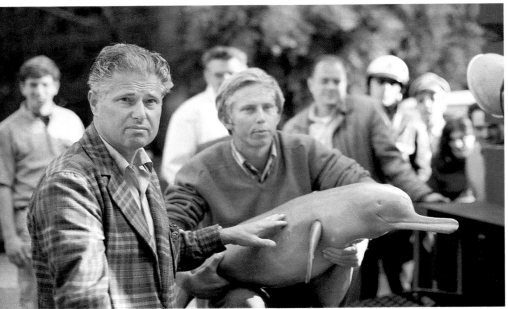

Figure 19. Steam-powered Khyber Express passing over the Rohri-Sukkur bridge at dusk. Built by the British in 1889, this iron bridge spans the Indus River.

Figure 20. Meeting the press at Steinhart Aquarium after being escorted by police from the airport. An exhausted Earl Herald and Bob Brownell display one of our dolphins during an impromptu press conference.

"They also study what happens if a person eats the poison. It is very bad. So, they take care."

The three young men who were doing the dissecting smiled and nodded. They were quick, but one had the impression that they were also very accurate. Elkan and I watched with a special intentness. It was no different from putting your life in the hands of an airline pilot, I said to myself.

"After three years, student fugu dissectors take a test," said the chamberlain. "When they pass, they must work as apprentice dissectors for a year. Then they get a license. It is all very careful."

Sure enough, after a day spent along the waterfront, our white-haired guide suggested that we repair to a "fugu house" for dinner. Since everything on the menu featured the potentially poisonous fish, even Earl and Bob had no alternatives.

We knelt on tatami mats around the low table, and awaited our fate. First the kimono-clad waitress brought a vase-like carafe of very hot sake, in which dried fugu fins had been allowed to steep. We watched silently as the five cups were filled with the amber liquid. Our host raised his glass, smiled and nodded at the assembled company, and drank deeply. We all followed suit.

The waitress reappeared with a tray of fugu sashimi, small pieces of raw, thinly-sliced fish. These were accompanied by a variety of exquisite sauces, for dipping.

This was followed by a course of cooked fugu. Between each course our cups were replenished with the hot sake, with its now-dissolved content of tetrodotoxin.

I found myself feeling more and more relaxed as we sat around the low table. It was warm and comfortable. The colors of the room were very agreeable. I had not noticed at first how colorful it was. And there were those flashes of color — now red, now yellow, now electric green and blue, as we sat talking. It was a wonderful evening. There was nothing to worry about — today, tomorrow, or ever.

Much later, the black sedan delivered us to our hotel.

I awoke the next morning without any trace of a hangover. The sense of peace and well-being lingered. As I lay in bed and looked around, I realized that I must have removed my contact lenses the night before, though I had no recollection of doing so.

Later, when I compared notes with Bob, Elkan and Earl, we discovered that we all had experienced similar sensations during the memorable fugu feast. A sense of complete relaxation, along with a continued awareness of our surroundings, and the hallucinatory flashes of bright color. We began to understand why the fugu is so popular.

I was invited to visit the reptile exhibit at the Ueno Park Zoo. I was excited about this, for the zoo is one of the few in the world boasting a pair of Komodo "dragons." These are very large monitor lizards, native to a small handful of islands in Indonesia. The lizards are rare, and only a limited number are allowed to be captured and sent to zoos.

A large Komodo dragon can reach ten feet in length, and weigh well over one hundred pounds. (Hence the name "dragon.") They are carnivores, and eat animals as large as goats and cattle, and carrion. They also appear to have remarkable intelligence, for a reptile.

There have been several well-documented cases of Komodo dragon attacks on humans. Bites by these lizards are especially dangerous, since great chunks of tissue can be lost to their sharp, recurved teeth, and because their mouths are populated with some highly virulent bacteria. Most human deaths from Komodo monitor bites have been related to fulminating infections.

At the Ueno Park Zoo, I was met by a Japanese veterinarian. He had only a few words of English, and I had only a few of Japanese, but our mutual interest in herpetology bridged the gap, and small talk was unnecessary.

The two Komodo dragons were housed in a large glassed-in cage with a concrete floor. There was a shallow pool, and some logs strewn about. A small door in the concrete wall was the only entrance.

The two lizards were young adults, each about seven-and-a-half feet long. They watched us unblinking, as my colleague and I stood looking through the glass.

The Japanese veterinarian gestured to the tiny door — would I like to go in with the lizards? I nodded, and followed him to this Alice-in-Wonderland-sized door. A keeper stood beside it as I ducked and followed my colleague into the enclosure.

I had barely time to straighten up and take one step forward, when there was a loud hiss, and the two dragons were bearing down on us.

My host was about five feet three inches tall; I am a foot taller. Wasting no time on "after you" protocol, I dove horizontally through the low doorway, knocking the door violently against the outside wall. The waiting keeper seized the door just in time to keep it from rebounding into the face of the other veterinarian, who was by now air-borne through the exit. The door was slammed in the leading dragon's angry, open-mouthed face.

My Japanese colleague and I picked ourselves up and dusted off. He smiled gamely, and the keeper burst into high-pitched, inscrutable oriental laughter.

"Now — drink?" said my fellow scientist, raising his hand to his mouth expressively.

"Yes," I nodded, still somewhat shaken.

We repaired to a nearby cafe, where we restored our equilibrium and our shattered egos with several locally brewed beers, and rice crackers.

I was now entitled to wear a Komodo dragon's tooth set in gold in my lapel. This distinction is reserved for those hardy (foolish) few who have survived an attack by a Komodo dragon. Fortunately, my colleague and I had no scars or lost organs to validate our claims. (Much later, on a visit to the National Zoo in Washington, DC, I was given three Komodo dragon teeth, one of which I had set into a gold lapel pin.)

Our group also made side trips to Enoshima and Aburatsubo, where there are outstanding exhibits of fishes, marine invertebrates, and aquatic mammals. The Japanese have pioneered many novel techniques for exhibiting these. In Enoshima, we saw a display of white mice living in an underwater container in an aquarium. A semi-permeable membrane allowed free diffusion of oxygen and carbon dioxide to and from the air-breathing rodents and their aquatic surroundings.

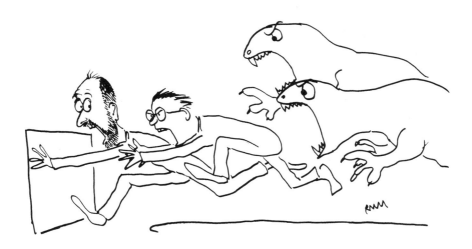

At Aburatsubo we saw a unique, doughnut-shaped tank. Visitors stand in the center and the fish swim around them, in a novel reversal of roles. Our chief, Earl Herald, took a keen interest in this, and later a similar, smaller tank was built at Steinhart Aquarium. (The design problems inherent in such a structure can only be imagined. There are no visible supports, the closely fitting glass panels must form a circle, and yet be water-tight. A miracle of engineering!)

The Japanese had also successfully confined and even bred many aquatic species that at that time had eluded the efforts of scientists in other parts of the world. We saw rare fishes, walruses, dolphins, and many small whales, thriving in their captive surroundings.

Just before we left Tokyo, Elkan and I, as the official photographers of the expedition, visited the city's camera supply centers. The exchange rate at the time was 360 yen to the dollar, and the two of us did all we could to boost the local economy. I bought a superb Nikon camera body, and a selection of lenses. I had been a photography buff for years, and had brought my trusty but noisy and cumbersome Exacta system with me on the trip. I decided to ship these home, and rely on the lighter and superior Nikon equipment.

(As it turned out, my confidence was well-placed. The camera endured the steamy climates of the Philippines, Thailand, and India, and two raging dust storms in Pakistan. None of my film was scratched, and back in San Francisco, when I submitted the camera for cleaning under the factory warranty, no internal cleaning was necessary. The well-fitted body and lenses had withstood even the blowing sands on the banks of the Indus.)

Before leaving Japan, we made arrangements with our colleagues at the University of Tokyo to provide short-term housing for any dolphins we might be bringing back, before our long return flight to San Francisco. The faculty and graduate students were happy to oblige.

We flew from Tokyo to Manila. As before, we were greeted with the familiar message discouraging us to go any farther. We shrugged this off with the ease of hardened criminals, and went about fulfilling our official duties in the Philippines.

Earl had been asked by the FAO to observe aquaculture and mariculture projects, and give advice. As it turned out, we learned more than we contributed.

The local experts had devised a system of shallow fresh water ponds, in which a small common fish, *Talapia*, happily converted unappetizing algae into edible fish protein. The fish were periodically harvested and sun dried, after which many of them were ground into a protein- and calcium-rich fish flour. When mixed with the locally milled rice flour or wheat flour, this *Talapia* flour greatly boosted the nutritional value of the native diet.

We sampled the native food at a sumptuous state dinner hosted by President and Madame Ferdinand Marcos, but I doubt that the plebeian *Talapia* fish flour figured in the menu. Elkan and I had no qualms about consuming everything that was set before us.

Ignoring official "advice," we flew on to Thailand. Kasetsart University, outside Bangkok, is the home of the famous preserved fish collection Earl was to inspect. Years before, the Vanderbilt Foundation had funded the gathering, preservation and maintenance of this collection of Southeast Asian fishes.

While Earl fulfilled his official duties, the rest of us were free to go sightseeing. I was eager to visit the Thai Red Cross's Venom Institute, where antivenins are produced for the treatment of poisonous snakebites. Bob and Elkan agreed to accompany me on this jaunt.

The snakes are kept in outdoor pits. These are sunk in the ground about two feet, and surrounded by a three-foot wall.

"My God!" said Elkan, as we gazed into one of these.

There were low shrubs growing in the pit, and festooned on and around these were hundreds of olive green and brown snakes, their sleek bodies glistening in the sunshine. Never had I seen so many cobras in one place.

"I thought snake pits only existed in horror movies and stories," said Bob.

I knew just what he meant. (The hero and villain wrestle on the brink; the villain finally topples in, with a blood-curdling cry, and dies an appalling death amidst the hissing serpents.)

As we gazed into the writhing pits at the Institute, it did not take a vivid imagination to see how easy it would be to accidentally fall in. Death would be swift and certain.

"How do they get them out, and get the venom out?" Bob wanted to know.

"We use tongs or snake hooks," said our guide. "We restrain the snake and milk the venom out. We have thousands of them here."

After the venom is extracted from the snakes, it is purified by freeze-drying. Then it is inoculated in gradually increasing doses into horses. As a horse develops an immunity to a specific venom, blood is drawn from it, at intervals of about eight to ten weeks. This blood is treated to isolate that portion containing the venom antibodies. This in turn is divided into individual doses, freeze-dried, and sealed into glass ampules. The antivenin produced by the Thai Red Cross's Venom Institute is distributed throughout the world.

The evening before we left Bangkok, we were the guests of the military junta in Thailand at a sumptuous banquet. Between the numerous courses, there were performances by the traditional Thai dancers.

Elkan and I remained fairly cheerful through the first several courses, which included birds' nest soup (Bob and Earl blanched visibly) and other mysterious and highly spiced dishes. I have a particular fondness for fiery hot peppers, and was approaching Nirvana.

Eventually a platter arrived before us that caused Elkan and me to hesitate. The contents were greyish-black, slightly gelatinous objects that gave off a sulfurous, foul odor.

"Ah, what it this?" I said, with forced heartiness.

"Great delicacy," said one of our hosts. "Thousand-year-old eggs."

Elkan and I exchanged glances.

"Really?" said Elkan affably. "Are they truly a thousand years old?"

"Not truly," said our host, smiling broadly. "But they have been buried in mud for a long, long time."

This I could believe! They were like oval mummies, only not so well preserved.

I took a deep breath. "Well, I've never tasted a thousand-year-old egg before!" And I courageously took one, and bit into it.

Elkan, watching me, followed suit. Earl and Bob looked the other way, intent on their lemon-grass-flavored prawns.

The taste was incredibly foul (no pun intended!) but I managed to swallow it. We got through the rest of the banquet, but later that night, I found myself collecting the wages of sin against my alimentary system.

My entire belly was bloated and tender. When I could manage it, I belched sulfurous gas. At one point during that endless night, Elkan knocked on the door between our two rooms.

"You okay, Fred?" he called. "It doesn't sound good in there."

"Doesn't smell good, you mean, maybe?" I said bitterly, rummaging in the tackle boxes for some source of relief.

"Well, I wasn't going to say so," said Elkan politely.

"Just don't light any matches," I said acrimoniously. "There'd be one hell of an explosion!"

"Must've been the eggs," Elkan said consolingly.

"And you still feel okay?" I said suspiciously.

"Yeah, I'm okay."

"Hmph."

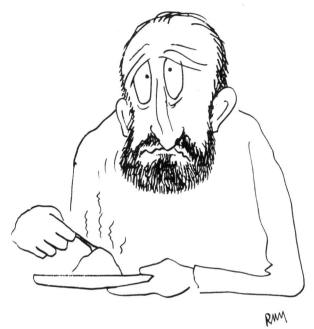

Thousand-year-old eggs. *Foul* tasting!

(After all this time has elapsed, I still cannot exorcise the suspicion that Elkan palmed *his* portion of the infamous eggs. He remained the picture of robust health.)

In the morning, we departed for Rangoon. My tourist experiences of that city, and of New Delhi, were limited to frequent visits to their toilet facilities. I was loath to visit these places in the first place, but afraid *not* to in the second!

When we arrived in Pakistan, I was beginning to feel better. (It is said that no western visitor can survive the first twenty-four hours in Karachi without developing "Karachi tummy;" I *arrived* with it!) However, my bout with the "thousand-year-old" eggs apparently immunized me against further gastrointestinal upsets. In the ensuing weeks, Earl, Bob and Elkan each had their trials, but I remained healthy. Perhaps those loathesome eggs should be analyzed for their medicinal properties!

Shortly after we checked into the Karachi Intercontinental Hotel, we received a summons to present ourselves at the American Consul-General's office. The weather was hot and oppressive, and Earl, despite his careful eating, was beginning to feel the first effects of dysentery. Nonetheless, we squared ourselves for the inevitable showdown. We had been told not to come; we had come. In fact, we had come halfway around the world, on a mission funded by the U.S. Navy, and we were not about to abandon it.

At the Consul-General's office, we were summoned to the office of the First Secretary. (Later, we were to learn that this unpleasant person was a CIA officer. Clearly, he had not been schooled in diplomacy.)

"You guys have your nerve, coming here," he said to Earl, as Elkan, Bob and I stood in the background.

"You were told not to come. In Hawaii. In Japan. In the Philippines, in Thailand." He ticked these places off on his thick fingers. "You've ignored the instructions of the United States government."

"We have received no explanations, no clarifications," said Earl patiently. "I've repeatedly requested these, and have received none."

"You don't need explanations! Just take my word for it!" He thumped his broad chest. "This place is *trouble* right now. You guys" — he shook his finger menacingly — "come along with your cameras and electronic equipment, and think you can go nosing around up the river. You could get in a lot of trouble! Cause *me* a lot of trouble!"

"Electronic equipment?" said Earl, with visible restraint. "What electronic equipment?"

"I know you have radios and tape recorders!" he said triumphantly. "They've been seen at the customs checks."

"A small cassette recorder, yes," said Earl. "It's for taking field notes. For our scientific study. The radio is Dr. Frye's small transistorized short wave set." He smiled grimly. "So we can hear the results of the U.S. presidential election." (It was Humphrey vs. Nixon; we had voted by absentee ballot before leaving home.)

"You were instructed not to come!" said the First Secretary, who was rapidly becoming purple. "You don't question a Telex message from your govenment — you just obey it!"

"But the government approved this expedition," said Earl. "The funding comes from the Navy. And the West Pakistani government invited us."

The veins on the man's temples were throbbing, and his face had become the color of a ripe satsuma plum.

"What the hell are you guys *really* here for?" he screamed at Earl, shaking his fist.

"I've told you," said Earl, who was starting to look hot and tired. "It's a scientific expedition, funded by the U.S. Navy, through the Smithsonian Institution, to the California Academy of Sciences. We were invited by the Pakistani government to study the blind dolphins of the Indus, and to bring some back with us."

"Dolphins!" shouted the fellow in obvious disbelief. "Well let me tell you this! You'd better not leave this city without specific permission from the Consul-General. And he's not available right now."

"We don't have unlimited time for this expedition," said Earl. "We have obligations back in the States by the end of November."

"Scientists!" sneered this miscast diplomat. "You guys don't know which end is up! Anybody who'd have the nerve to come here after being told not to!"

With this parting bit of bravado, he waved us from his presence.

After this unpleasant interlude, we made contact with Cedric Watson, the former British Army officer who was to lead our expedition up the Indus. Watson was in his late forties, blue-eyed and sandy-haired, with a straight back and firm step, no doubt instilled in him at Sandhurst Military Academy, where he had concluded his education. He was, in fact, part Pakistani, and a Pakistani citizen. However, his Pakistani forbears were obviously outnumbered by his English ones, and in appearance, speech and bearing he seemed the archetypal British military man. He was obviously accustomed to commanding, and to being obeyed.

We met with Watson at our hotel, where we gathered in Earl's suite to discuss the situation.

"They might put us under surveillance here at the hotel, and actively prevent us from leaving the city," said Earl, who was looking tired.

"Rubbish!" said Watson briskly. "They haven't placed you under house arrest, merely warned and advised. Still, it might not be a bad idea to give them the slip."

With military precision, Cedric Watson organized a plan for "giving them the slip." The following evening, his Land Rover and pickup truck were parked near the service door behind the hotel's kitchen. Natives in his employ gradually and discreetly brought down our gear and stowed it away. Then these men slipped into our rooms to "replace" us, and to make appropriate noises with drawers and plumbing in case we were under surveillance. Meanwhile, one by one, we strolled down to the dining room, as though for a late evening snack. Then, unobserved, we each slipped into the kitchen, and out the back into the waiting vehicles.

Bob was the last to come, and as we waited in the darkness, it seemed an eternity before he appeared, moving quickly to join Elkan and me in the back seat.

"Right!" said Cedric Watson in his clipped tones. "We're off." He started the engine, and guided the Land Rover out into the traffic. Behind us, the lights of the pickup truck followed closely.

We threaded our way out of the city, and took the road northeast, which follows the course of the Indus. As we drove through the darkness, Cedric told us about the country and the people.

"We should reach the twin cities of Rohri and Sukkur by early afternoon," he said, "if we don't have too many flats. We'll take time off on the way to visit the fortified palace at Kot Digi. It's quite remarkable."

"At Rohri and Sukkur we'll leave the vehicles. A fellow will be there to meet us with some boats. He's recruited a number of boys from the local people to work for us. You'll each have your own batman."

"Do you think that's necessary?" said Earl. "We're not used to being waited on."

"They're very useful," said Cedric. "And it gives employment to more people. It's what they expect."

"I'll feel like a colonial imperialist!" I quipped.

"I could get used to it," said Elkan, musingly. "But what about going home again? My wife's not going to wait on me hand and foot. It could be a real culture shock!"

"I'm willing to risk it," said Bob, the only one of us who was not married.

Cedric listened in tolerant silence to this Yankee exchange.

We passed through the city of Hyderabad around dawn. We had been dozing, but Cedric was as alert and upright as ever. During World War II he had commanded a small British warship in the Indian Ocean.

As soon as the sun came up, the temperature began to rise. Although this was October, the average midday temperature was one hundred and twenty degrees.

We were driving along the hot, uneven pavement when the truck behind us scunded three short blasts on the horn.

"Ah!" said Cedric, glancing in the rearview mirror. "Our first flat. We may as well stretch our legs. Would you care for some tea? I have a thermos."

We stood in the blazing sun as the native driver changed the tire. It was our first experience in being waited on, and in that heat, we were glad just to watch.

A few miles down the road, Cedric pulled up at a decrepit "garage" — a shack and a mud brick oven. A peeling sign in Urdu script proclaimed the owner's line of business.

"You chaps might like to watch this," Cedric said. "I daresay you do it differently in the States."

Getting out, he addressed the elderly proprietor in fluent Urdu. The native driver gave the old Sindhi the flat tire, and he carried it into the shade of his workshop. The tube had already been patched many times. The old man squatted on the floor, threaded a straight sewing needle, and stitched the rent with a baseball-like stitch.

Next he took a gourd from his work bench, and stirred the contents with a stick.

"Raw rubber gum," said Cedric, who must have watched this procedure many times before. The old Sindhi daubed this over the site of the repair, and placed over it a graft cut from an expired tube, hanging from a nail on the wall. Then, trotting out to the mud brick oven, he returned with a hot iron.

"Heated with camels' dung," said Cedric conversationally.

Using the hot iron, the old man vulcanized the patch onto the tube. Then, with many smiles and nods of his turbaned head, he attached an ancient bicycle pump to the valve, and pumped vigorously until the tire and tube were inflated again. We were ready to roll.

That patch held up for a good twenty miles of hot, uneven pavement, before it went out again!

Some time later, Cedric pointed ahead. "There's the fortified palace at Kot Digi." Rising from the plain was a large sandstone and mud brick edifice, with crenelated battlements.

"I thought you said it was hundreds of years old," said Bob. "It looks brand new!"

Cedric chuckled. "It is well-preserved, isn't it? Because it's so confoundedly dry here. No rain to melt the bricks, or rot the wood. Across the road are much more ancient Harappan ruins, going back five thousand years. They've been under excavation for years. There's always some archeological team or other camped about."

We got out at the fortified castle, and walked around. In one wall were massive double doors, studded with sharp iron spikes.

"Pretty intimidating," said Elkan. "Doesn't look like you could get in without an invitation."

We climbed the stairs to some of the cell-like rooms in the upper stories, and looked out through the arched windows over the Indus floodplain. Below, in one of the courtyards, was a brick-lined well that appeared to be still functioning.

In the harem quarters, Cedric pointed to some wooden lattice screens. "These were to keep unauthorized people from seeing the women. See how intricately they're put together, without any metal hardware." Looking up, we saw painted flowers and birds on the plastered ceiling, their colors still bright.

When we had seen and photographed the sights of Kot Digi, we got back in the Land Rover.

"We should be in Rohri and Sukkur by one o'clock," Cedric said. "The river runs east and west at that point. Rohri is on the south bank, Sukkur is on the north. They are linked by an old railroad bridge. A steam train runs back and forth between the two. You Americans don't have many steam trains, do you?"

"Only short runs, as tourist attractions," I said.

"Disneyland," murmured Bob.

"Well, you may get a crack at riding the old Khyber Express. If we're successful in capturing some *buhlaan*, as the natives call dolphins, it would probably be best to bring them back to Karachi by train. It's not an 'express' in the European sense of the word, but there's no risk of flat tires. In this heat, it would be wise."

We arrived at Rohri and Sukkur shortly after noon. As arranged, two small dhow-like boats were there to meet us, manned by several native young men. When our gear was transferred to these, the truck and Land Rover were consigned to the care of a dark-skinned young boy. Cedric addressed him in swift Urdu. We could not understand the words, but the tone was definitely menacing. Clearly, the vehicles had better be just as we left them, or else!

The two boats were fitted with ragged lateen-type sails, and long sweep oars aft. Our destination was about eight miles upriver, against the sluggish current.

"Now we're leaving the province of Sind, and moving into Baluchistan," said Cedric, as we set out. Earl and I were in the first boat with him.

"These people are Baluchis, for the most part. Moslems, of course. Many of them have four wives, as permitted by the Koran. This fellow" — he nodded at the young man plying the oars — "is the son of the local tribal headman. There's no village, so to speak, but a collection of boats which congregate here and there. A few people upriver have some reed huts and cultivate crops, but most of them live on the river."

The wind was only a light breeze; our progress was slow. Shouting back to his cohorts in the second boat, the headman's son took the end of a handmade hemp rope attached to the bow, and jumped overboard. He swam the short distance to shore, and began towing us upstream.

Looking back at the second boat, we could see Elkan struggling with a blanket, which he was rigging as an auxiliary sail. Bob held it as he tied it in place. The tribesmen watched this procedure with interest. However, this did little to augment the boat's progress, and soon it, too, was being towed.

We continued in this style, sometimes broken by interludes of wind, or with someone at the oars, until we reached our campsite on the western bank of the river, about midafternoon.

A throng of native men greeted us, and began unloading the gear. The boats and families of some of these could be seen not far away.

As promised, each of us had a personal batman, who pitched our tents, and brought us tea. The batman is a holdover from the English colonial system, and dates to their halcyon days of Nineteenth Century imperialism. In the mornings, these servants would offer to shave us, and to polish our boots, should any of us wish to wear shiny boots while prowling around the floodplain of western Baluchistan! As for the shaving, we were not comfortable with this, and with the exception of Earl, we all grew beards during our time in camp.

My personal batman was a native Pakistani, but unlike the others, he was an English-speaking Christian. His name was Victor Nathaniel, and he was a veterinarian, a graduate of the University of Lahore, in the north. Veterinary positions were hard to come by, and he had taken this menial job as batman in Cedric's expedition.

Victor was polite, but did not fraternize with us. He would speak when spoken to, but never volunteered anything in the group. Had he done so, I sensed, he would quickly have been "put in his place" by Watson.

Cedric was undeniably an autocrat. He was the product of a society built on the class system. British rule had ended several decades before, but Cedric, presumably capitalizing on his Pakistani lineage and citizenship, enjoyed the best of the old world and the new. He and his British wife lived on a plantation southeast of Karachi.

The real power in Pakistan, we came to understand, was wielded by the wealthy. In this oligarchy, a small percentage of the people reportedly held eighty to ninety percent of the wealth. We did not doubt that Cedric belonged to this favored group. True, he did run his business of collecting animals for zoos, but this seemed more a gentleman's hobby than an urgent means of survival.

Our camp was about thirty yards from the river. The only shade was provided by our tents, and these became stifling during the hottest part of the day. A thicket of scrubby acacia and tamarind trees bordered the camp, but provided no real shade.

A cadaverous-looking native man was in charge of the cooking. His name was Ramsan, and his chronic cough was the first thing I heard every morning.

The camp was astir at dawn every day, although none of the native men had timepieces. I watched, fascinated, their early morning ablutions. Each man would stroll to the nearby thicket and select a tamarind twig, which he would chew until one end was flattened and frayed. This was used to brush the teeth. Next, he would use the twig to tickle the back of his throat, to induce a gag reflex. The night's accumulation of phlegm was spat out. Following this, the same twig was used to clean each nostril. Finally, the unfrayed end of the stick was used to clean the ear canals.

Then, going over to the river, the man would wash his face, hands, and feet. Putting his shoes back on, he was then ready to kneel in the direction of Mecca, and say the first of the five daily prayers.

The Koran forbids touching the lips to tobacco, but the camp boys had a way around this. When they could obtain cigarettes from Cedric, they would hold them between the third and fourth fingers of the right hand (the left hand being "unclean" in the Moslem faith), and cup the hand into a circular cone. Then, by placing their lips on the opening between the thumb and forefinger, they could draw smoke from the cigarette. (Such ingenuity in finding a "loophole" in the Moslem law is worthy of our wiliest lawyers, who have to go to school to learn the technique!)

Most of the camp boys were native Baluchis or Sindhis, although there was one, our "snake man," who was a Joghi. The Joghis are descendents of the original gypsy tribes, which originated in Western Hindustan. The Joghis are at the bottom of the social class system. Those we saw were always ragged, with tattered turbans. This young man was a cocky but somewhat indolent fellow, the son of the chieftain of a nearby Joghi enclave.

We hoped to bring back some cobras and other native snakes, and it was the job of this Joghi to search these out, capture them, and bring them back to camp. By the time we were ready to return home, we had several cobras, sand vipers, sand boas and assorted lizards and turtles.

The morning of our second day in camp, we were seated around the folding table, drinking tea and finishing off our breakfast of eggs and chapatis. Suddenly Cedric stopped chewing and raised his head, listening.

"Listen!" he said, and we all stopped eating. The day was clear, and already warm. In the distance, coming from the south, we could hear a faint droning — the sound made by a single-engine plane.

"A plane!" exclaimed Cedric. "You never see a plane around here! Who the hell —?"

Then, as he looked at us, the light dawned. "Your friends in Karachi," he said ironically. "They must be checking up on you."

We all rose from the table, looking hurriedly around at the tents and the crates of equipment. We would have liked to camouflage them, but there was no time.

"Into the thicket!" said Cedric, in his most military tones. He barked a few short orders in Urdu to the native boys, who were looking at the southern sky and pointing excitedly.

Feeling a little foolish, but also very excited, we all scurried into the bushes, where we crouched and watched the approach of the plane.

The plane flew low over the campsite, continued northward for a half mile, and then swung around and flew over the camp a second time.

"Checking us out, all right," said Cedric, with grim satisfaction. "An old Piper Cub. They must have flown up from Karachi or Hyderabad,"

"What do they expect to see," said Bob, "a military training camp?"

"That's it," I agreed. "We're really training all these fellows in hand-to-hand combat and other secret techniques, known only to ourselves."

"It's that chess set you brought along," said Elkan. "I saw you teaching your batman to play last evening. We all know it's really a military strategy teaching tool. You should have known it would not go undetected!"

We all laughed gleefully, looking up at the circling plane from our shelter in the bushes, and feeling like a bunch of kids playing hide and seek. Or cops and robbers. The thing was, we were neither cops nor robbers. Simply good guys (relatively) trying to do a job.

After about fifteen minutes of circling our camp, the plane headed south, from whence it had come.

"I hope they're satisfied," said Cedric, as we came out of hiding, laughing and picking leaves and thorns from our clothes.

A few days later, we moved our camp up river a few miles, where we remained for the rest of our stay.

As the medical officer of the group, I felt responsible for the wholesomeness of the food served us. The cook's chronic cough, I suspected, was the result of tuberculosis. Also, our water supply — the river — was shared with a herd of water buffalo upstream, and also jackals, wild dogs, and other animals.

With my batman, Victor, as translator, I tried to impress on Ramsan the necessity for boiling all water and utensils, and for washing his own hands with soap. I gave him a bar of Dial soap from my own supplies.

Ramsan listened and nodded, but as though he were catering to a whim. Who on earth would want boiling water when the midday temperature was one hundred and twenty degrees? When he boiled it and set it to cool, the water would only really begin to cool late at night, when the temperature dropped to around fifty-five degrees. Thus, in order for us to have even tepid, safe drinking water, the cook had to boil it a day in advance.

The days were roasting hot, and as a result, we became a bit lax about drinking only boiled water or tea. Later, I was to pay dearly for this lapse.

A staple of our menu was chapatis, chewy, unleavened flat bread that was baked on the clay firepot. The first wife of the headman was in charge of these. About an hour before the meal, she would mix wheat flour and water into a large ball of dough, which she kneaded assiduously. She would pinch off lemon-sized portions from this and flatten them with her palms and fingertips. When these were baked and served hot, they were delicious. The natives, who ate with their families, used chapatis as a spoon, which they dipped into the community pot.

Curried rice was another staple. For the rest, we alternated between ground camel meat, an occasional goat, and much "chicken" — a euphemism for the tough and stringy semi-domesticated game fowl of the area. Often there was fish, or even turtle meat, caught by our Sindhi fisherman, Nathah. Some of the catfish weighed more than eighty pounds. Everything was eaten fresh because there was no refrigeration. There were never any leftovers since there were always plenty of mouths to consume these.

An itinerant confection merchant paddled up to our camp every few days with a tray full of sweets made from rice or squash. This old man was the object of much mischievous teasing by the camp boys. One would tweak his beard or his turban, and while his head was turned towards his tormentor, another would grab a handful of sweets. Eventually, the old man would weep pitiably and depart, only to return and subject himself to more abuse in a day or so.

Our diet was also augmented by occasional melons, cucumbers or tomatoes, bartered from a native patch. These were raised along the floodplain in trenches dug down to the water table, and filled with compost. Natural seepage provided an efficient irrigation system.

For breakfast, I was fond of spreading peanut butter on the warm chapatis, from my own private two-pound jar, imported lovingly from the U.S.A. (This, too, must have been noted at customs. How could anyone suspect anti-American motives from a man who travels with his own peanut butter?)

"How can you eat that stuff?" said Cedric, in friendly derision. "It looks like something out of a baby's nappy."

As he spoke, he was spreading *his* chapatis with his own particular favorite, rich brown apple butter.

"And that stuff?" I said, pointing an accusing finger.

"Apple butter?" he said in surprise. "It's not the same thing at all."

Cedric liked his soft-boiled eggs cooked exactly two minutes, so they were just nicely runny. One morning, while we were still getting dressed, we heard a commotion outside. Cedric's voice was raised in angry Urdu, and we heard snatches of Ramsan's voice, responding in a pitiful whine. We tumbled out of our tents to find Cedric holding his rifle pressed into the old cook's stomach.

"What's going on here?" said Earl sternly. Ramsan turned pleading eyes on us, while continuing to whine and wave his arms in the air.

"Dammit, I told this bloody idiot how I wanted my eggs!" said Cedric angrily, still holding the gun barrel against the old man's belly.

"And what do I get?" He gestured towards the table. "They're damned near hard boiled! Unfit for anything but the jackals!" He glared at the cook, who was cowering visibly.

"Now see here," said Earl. "That's not worth all this commotion. Put the gun away, and let's sit down and have tea while Ramsan cooks more eggs."

With one more threatening glare, Cedric pulled his rifle away, and stalked to his tent.

After a somewhat subdued breakfast, Cedric was once more restored to his urbane self.

The word was spread about to all the river people that the scientist-sahibs wanted some live buhlaan, as the dolphins were called locally. The buhlaan have been caught and used by these people for millennia. The meat is eaten in a variety of cooked dishes. The bones are carved into cooking utensils and combs. The thick blubber layer beneath the skin is rendered for oil. This is clarified and stored in jars, where it keeps a long time. It is used in clay lamps for lighting, for cooking, and as a hair dressing.

One day when I was out in a dugout canoe with Victor, we met an old fisherman, and fell to discussing the buhlaan. The old man made a long speech, and Victor turned to translate.

"He says buhlaan oil is very good for an old man like he is, married to four young wives. He says it helps him keep his wives happy."

The old man, watching my face, nodded and grinned a toothy smile. He broke into another long speech.

"He says the best oil for this is from the 'melon' on the forehead of the buhlaan. In case you would like to try it, sometime."

We thanked the old man for sharing his wisdom, and he paddled happily away.

The natives had two methods of capturing the dolphins. The simplest was to tether a small catfish alongside their boat, to lure the buhlaan in close. When this happened, a net was tossed over it, effectively entrapping it.

A second method involved locating the creatures, then laying down nets in nearby small bays and mouths of streams, and driving the dolphins into these. Canoe paddles were slapped on the water's surface in order to drive the dolphins into the nets.

Once we were established at our permanent camp, the camp boys set about digging a holding pool for any dolphins that might be captured. The task was fairly easy, in the fine sand of the floodplain. Once the water table was reached, water began to seep up from below. In two days, the pool was filled, and ready for occupancy.

Our days were spent paddling up and down the river, photographing the local people at work, and studying the local fauna. In addition to collecting snakes, I had acquired two hedgehogs, "Paki" and "Stan," which I hoped to ease home in a false bottom built into one of the wooden snake boxes. I doubted that any customs official would look beyond the cobra in the top compartment, if that far!

Often in our excursions on the river we would see natives on shore using stone implements. I had the opportunity to collect several flake knives, scrapers, and burins that were of contemporary origin. Most were made from chert or flint, which came from the region of the Afghanistan border.

I held "sick call' every afternoon at my tent. Not only was I the medical official for our immediate party, but also, as word spread, for any ailing members of the far-flung families of our camp personnel. This gave me an excellent opportunity to observe these people at close range.

The men, even those in late middle age, were a magnificent lot, with healthy teeth and well-muscled bodies. Even among men in their seventies, I saw no cases of cataract or glaucoma. (However, fly-borne trachoma was common among the Joghis, or gypsies.)

The women were another story. I saw no women beyond their mid-thirties, and these were prematurely aged, due to frequent pregnancy, prolonged nursing, and recurrent infections.

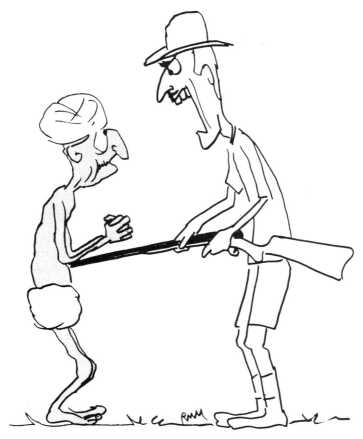

"Dammit, I told this idiot how I wanted my eggs!"

From earliest childhood, females are at a disadvantage in this society. Up and down the river, I noticed girl children surely less than two years old sitting on the bare ground with sisters and female cousins, performing small household tasks. Thus from infancy they were exposed to such parasites as hookworms and threadworms, which are easily transmitted through moist soil.

In contrast, male infants are pampered, nursed and carried, and allowed to play until early adolescence, when they start to learn masculine skills and the teachings of Mohammed.

When a young Baluchi girl reaches menarche, it is not unusual for her to be betrothed to a much older man, as his youngest wife. Because of the lack of health care and harsh climate, most women are in their prime in their late teen years, and within a decade are in declining health.

In my "clinic," all female patients were chaperoned by a male relative, either a husband or a son. It was taboo for me to conduct any personal examination, and all questions and answers were filtered through the male relative.

"Ask her where it hurts," I would say to Victor, who would translate to the son or husband, who alone could ask the woman these intimate questions. Her reply would come back in the same circuitous way.

One of my first patients was our chapati maker, first wife of the local headman, and mother of the young man who had towed us up river. A few weeks before our arrival, she had been scratched in both eyes while gathering firewood. Her corneas had been injured, and by the time we arrived she had lost much of her sight due to the proliferation of scar tissue over the corneas. I treated her eyes four times a day with antibiotic-corticosteroid ophthalmic ointment, and by the end of our stay, most of her vision had been restored.

One day when Victor and the headman and I were alone, I asked him a question that had intrigued me ever since we arrived.

"How do you manage to keep four wives happy, without jealousy?" I asked through Victor. I thought of the close quarters these people lived in, on their boats and in their huts on shore.

The headman, who was in his fifties, fixed me with laughing brown eyes, and a wry smile at the corners of his mouth. He made a short speech to Victor, and waited for him to translate.

"He says that his youngest wife is eighteen, and his oldest wife is thirty-three. It is easy, he says. He makes love to each one on the same night, and each thinks that she is the *only* one!"

The old man laughed, and Victor and I joined him.

In the evenings, the men would gather in our camp and perform on musical instruments, and dance. The instruments were the *be'en*, a twin-reed gourd flute, a drum, and occasionally, a native violin. The women were excluded from this entertainment; they congregated in another area for songs and gossip.

A group of people on the river who fascinated me were the "heron people." These natives spent most of their lives aboard small, double-ended boats, seldom measuring more than twenty feet long and six feet wide. They lived by fishing, which was done for them by tame herons, which they caught and trained.

Capturing live herons was a highly developed art with these people. The men had decoy hats, made from the cured skins of dead herons. The head and neck portions were stuffed and fixed upright; the body was formed into the tight-fitting cap. When worn by a hunter who was crouched in the shallow water, the decoys did look like living birds. An adept hunter could approach wild herons and seize their legs before they could escape.

Another technique was to tether a tame heron on a perch which protruded from a floating reed blind. When wild herons were attracted to the live decoy, their legs were grabbed from beneath the water.

The captured herons were hobbled with reed anklets, and attached to perches on the gunwales of the boat. They were tamed by being handfed, which made them dependent on humans. When they were tame enough to be worked without trying to escape, a ring of woven plant fiber was placed around their necks, and they were freed to retrieve fish for their masters. The necklace prevented the birds from swallowing their prey. They were fed small fish scraps, which they were able to swallow.

These birds were part of the family network crowded aboard each boat. Typically, there would be a man, one or more wives, his widowed mother, and numerous children. Cooking, eating and sleeping all were done in the tiny cabin made of saplings and woven reed matting. From time to time this would be dismantled and taken ashore, where it served as a shelter while the family foraged on land or repaired the vessel.

One day Victor and I were invited into one of these. It measured about six feet by eight feet, and the walls were decorated with photographs of Pakistani movie stars!

One morning I was crouched in a hastily constructed reed blind, hoping to photograph the heron people at work. As I waited, three

women walked into view. The youngest, about seventeen, was obviously pregnant. As the two older women eased her into a reclining
position on the sand, I realized that I was about to witness the birth
process.

I felt some pangs of conscience; they were obviously unaware of
my presence. But to stand up and announce myself would be very dis-
concerting to all concerned. I decided to stay put, but to refrain from
using my camera. I realized that if I were discovered, it might jeopar-
dize our whole expedition. Feeling like a voyeur, I watched the entire
birth process through my telephoto lens.

The girl rolled on her side, as labor progressed. One of the women
scooped a shallow hole in the sand and lined it with rags. The girl was
helped to a squatting position over the hole. Very quickly, and with
little outward signs of distress, she delivered her baby into the rag-
lined depression. The umbilical cord was severed with what appeared
to be a shard of glass or a stone blade.

The baby was wiped briskly dry with a rag, and introduced to its
mother's breast. Soon the placenta and a small quantity of blood were
passed through the birth canal, and buried in the hole.

About forty minutes after giving birth, the mother, with her new
infant slung on her back, returned to the melon field to resume her
work.

One afternoon some fishermen excitedly paddled to our camp with
three dolphins in tow. The creatures had been caught in nets, and now
were being towed behind the three dugout boats by means of lan-
yards tied around their beak-like jaws. These aquatic mammals
breathe through a blowhole on the top of the head, and fortunately,
had not been drowned in transit.

We paid the fishermen handsomely, and transferred the dolphins
to our riverside "holding tank." When the excitement had subsided
and we were free to examine them, we discovered that these "blind"
dolphins did possess small eyes, but that these rudimentary sight
organs were covered with skin. It is doubtful that these eyes can
discern anything beyond differences in light and dark.

We weighed each dolphin, measured it, and gave it an injection of
antibiotics and a cortisone-like drug to prevent infection and relieve
capture-induced stress. Each day we observed them, although the
water of our pool was as silt-laden as the river, and we could not clearly distinguish their swimming patterns. Part of our experiments involved taking water samples from different depths of the river to determine how much light was available to these creatures. We concluded that there was very little light, even near the surface.

While we were conducting our experiments at our riverside camp, we experienced two intense wind storms. The wind would pick up the fine sand of this alluvial plain and hurl it with fury over the landscape. Our tents withstood the blast, but even when we huddled in them at mealtime, the grit was in everything. I was wearing contact lenses (having lost my prescription sunglasses over the side of the canoe one day), and went around with my eyes screwed up to slits. The only casualty of the storm was our privy, four stakes in the ground surrounded by reed matting, which blew over most inopportunely for its hapless occupant!

One morning Elkan and I were taking pictures down by the buhlaan pool, when I noticed a particularly pretty girl about ten or eleven years old, looking suspiciously at us from her father's dugout canoe. I took a few pictures of her through my telephoto lens. She was dressed in rags, and had the obvious signs of a headlouse infestation.

"Tell her we'd like to see her and her mother," I said to Victor. When the mother and aunt approached us, I gave them a bar of Dial soap and a dose of insecticidal shampoo. Victor explained how these were to be used, and instructed them to bathe the young girl. Her name, we discovered, was Adjiani.

The mother and aunt immediately began scrubbing Adjiani. They dressed her in some clean, less ragged clothes, probably thinking that one of the sahibs wished to marry her.

Adjiani's transformation was remarkable. The previously suspicious and shy child was now warmly smiling at us, and dared to approach close enough to accept some candy. Elkan and I scrounged among our belongings and came up with some things we thought she and her family could use — a comb, a nail file, and a pocket mirror.

Adjiani's five-year-old sister approached, and asked if she, too, could have a bath with the sweet-smelling soap. Victor nodded, and she, too, received what was probably her first bath with soap.

"If their clothes weren't so ragged, they'd be beautiful children," Elkan said. "It's too bad their mother can't afford to dress them properly."

"Clothes can't be that expensive around here," I mused. "I'd be willing to donate a few rupees to the cause."

Elkan agreed, and hit Earl and Bob for donations too. We bestowed this small sum on the girls' mother, and Victor explained to her that it was for clothes for her daughters.

A few days later, we saw the two sisters again. They were dressed in their old rags, and Adjiani's hair showed the unmistakable signs of another louse infestation.

Later, when I got home to Berkeley and discussed the matter with Brucye, we tried to legally adopt Adjiani. However, we were stymied by the U.S. Department of State, for technical reasons. Adjiani and her sister were probably consigned to an older man as new wives as soon as they reached the age of twelve or thirteen, and by now, each is probably the mother of at least a half dozen children of her own. Brucye and I made donations to CARE on their behalf for ten years, hoping that at least *their* meager lives could be made a little easier. Adjiani's smiling, youthful, "before" and "after" photographs hang on the wall in my study.

After several weeks on the river bank, we began our preparations for transporting our precious live cargo back to San Francisco. We were able to obtain from Sukkur some old Lipton tea crates. These were dismantled, brought up river, and rebuilt into three appropriate shipping crates by our camp carpenter. We lined them with heavy-gauge plastic sheeting, brought from home.

A few days before our planned departure, we tested the dolphins' response to these shipping crates. When they were placed in ten inches of water in the boxes, they floundered about and nearly drowned. We finally settled on covering each buhlaan with moist T-shirt material, to keep them cool and prevent the delicate skin from drying.

The buhlaan were the final things to be packed when we broke camp on the last day. We made the boat trip down to Sukkur in good time, and found the vehicles as we had left them.

When the animals and gear were loaded in the pickup truck, it immediately became mired in the soft sand. Cool under pressure, Cedric summoned a nearby team of yoked oxen, who pulled the vehicle free.

We made it to the train station with little time to spare, and saw our precious cargo safely stowed aboard. We bade a temporary farewell to Cedric, who would be driving down to Karachi with his vehicles and the men he had brought from his plantation.

The Khyber Express was certainly not an "express" as we understand the word. (Compared to a yoke of oxen, though, it was quite fast.) The coal-burning, wooden-coached relic stopped every few minutes, it seemed, and took nineteen hours to reach Karachi, 515 kilometers away.

"When we get back to civilization, you fellows really must shave," said Earl as we trundled along in the heat. "Those beards are inappropriate for scientists, especially when we stop in Tokyo and see our colleagues at the University."

Before we had time to shave, though, we were set upon by the First Secretary from the American Consulate.

"I could have you arrested and deported as Class 3-C prisoners!" he said threateningly.

"What's that?" Bob murmured in my ear.

"Felons arrested for heinous crimes against the state," I grinned. We were all feeling frisky and independent, having succeeded in our mission beyond our wildest expectations.

"Which state, I wonder?" said Bob from behind his beard.

The First Secretary postured and threatened for a few more minutes, and then, apparently feeling he had fulfilled his duty, let us go.

We left our three dolphins in a fish pond at the home of the Pan American Airways agent, where his young daughter graciously donated her goldfish for their meal.

We retired to the Karachi International Hotel for a hot shower, and a good night's rest. The next morning we boarded a Boeing 707 and began our long journey home. The dolphins were the last passengers to board and the first to exit at every stop along the way. At our stops in New Delhi, Calcutta and Hong Kong there was at least a child's-size wading pool filled with tepid water for our peripatetic porpoises.

In Tokyo, they were trucked to a swimming tank, where they were allowed to swim undisturbed for sixteen hours. During that time they were watched over by graduate students from the University of Tokyo, while we ate and slept.

At San Francisco International Airport, a police escort eased our way through the traffic to Golden Gate Park, and the Steinhart Aquarium.

It was only when we were able to observe the dolphins in clear water that we learned that they swim on their sides. They rise to the surface, take in air, and then roll over on their right sides, moving their heads back and forth in a sweeping motion.

We later learned that while thus moving their heads, the dolphins emit an almost continuous stream of pulsed, high-frequency sounds. Tape recordings of these revealed that the animals were capable of discriminating underwater objects with unheard-of accuracy.

Anatomical studies of the head, especially the "melon," revealed the mechanism of this bio-sonar. The rounded area of the head functions as an acoustic lens, which focuses the sound waves. These are sent outward in a forward direction, creating a wedge-shaped "beam." Echoes returning from fixed and moving objects are received and transduced by the melon before they are processed by the dolphin's brain.

It was not until we returned to San Francisco that we learned of the attempted assassination of General Mohammad Ayub Khan, President of West Pakistan. This had occurred while we were camped on the river.

It appears that our CIA, while probably not involved in the matter, was aware that a *coup d'etat* was a distinct possibility at that time. Our presence in that sensitive area could have been misinterpreted by friend and foe alike. Undoubtedly, had we been approached more openly and diplomatically, we would have been more receptive to changing our plans.

All of these events had their consequences. Our visas for Pakistan were not to be renewed, by an edict from our own Department of State. The First Secretary in Karachi, we learned later, was posted to another duty station. And Cedric Watson, after the attempted assassination, wisely changed his name to that of one of his Pakistani forbears.

Elkan's movie of our adventures was never made. Most of his ten thousand feet of film become overheated during our slow trip on the Khyber Express, and was ruined. Thus my still photographs became the official record of our memorable expedition to the Indus.

8 | Back in Berkeley

"Festus" was a black and white cat that was boarded at our hospital. Most animals were boarded for a few days or a few weeks, while their owners were on vacation. Festus had been at the Berkeley Dog & Cat Hospital for four years when my partner and I bought the establishment.

Festus's owner, Mrs. Riley, came by twice a week to visit her cat. She was a large, middle-aged woman, with a stoic air. She would hold the cat on her lap and stroke it, silently.

Her husband hated cats. When she had first brought Festus home, he had forbidden her to keep the creature. It was then that she had hit upon the idea of boarding the cat nearby, and paying for it out of her household budget.

Mrs. Riley was a woman of infinite patience. For six years she made her twice weekly visit, and paid her boarding bill promptly. Then, for the next three years, her visits were less frequent, although the boarding check still came like clockwork. Her time was taken up with her ailing husband.

Finally, nine years after the once-young cat had been brought in, Mrs. Riley telephoned.

"I'll be coming in to bring Festus home tomorrow," she said. "My husband died last week. Now that the wake is over, I'm ready to bring my cat home."

All of us on the staff appreciated the momentousness of the occasion. *Nine years* these two had waited to be reunited! Festus was groomed with care.

123

Mrs. Riley arrived on the dot of 2:00. She was wearing a new print dress, and had a spot of rouge on each cheek.

"I'm having some friends in this afternoon," she said excitedly, "to help me welcome my baby home. A nice quiet ladies' tea, with a saucer of milk for His Highness."

We all gathered in the reception room as the cat was put in its carrier, and the pair left. Festus had been at the hospital longer than any of us.

Festus's homecoming party was recounted to us later by one of Mrs. Riley's friends. As the ladies sat drinking their tea, Festus was held in his mistress's lap. Suddenly, as she was caressing him, he sank his teeth into her wrist, leaped down, and dashed through an open French door. Her last sight of him was as he streaked through the yard, running.

Beowulf and Inga were a magnificent pair of Siberian Huskies. They were brother and sister, having been chosen from the same litter by two young clients of mine. The young people came by the hospital for advice.

"Inga has just come into heat for the first time, and we'd like to breed her," Greg said, "though not to Beowulf, of course." Amy giggled.

"We'd like to get Beowulf fixed, but we don't want him to become sluggish and fat. What do you think?"

I suggested a vasectomy, which would render the dog sterile, but otherwise keep his masculinity intact. The couple agreed, and I kept Beowulf overnight, and performed the surgery the next day.

The following day, Greg and Amy called for their dog.

"Beowulf may still be a bit sore, and probably won't try anything athletic," I cautioned, "but you'd better keep him away from Inga as long as she's still in heat. It'll be six weeks before he's completely sterile."

An hour later, I had a distraught phone call from Amy. "Beowulf got away from us when we got home, and he — uh — well — he *did it* with Inga."

"Well, I could give her an injection that would assure she doesn't get pregnant, but there are side effects," I said. "You might not want to risk it."

I held the line while there was a muffled consultation on the other end.

"Dr. Frye? Okay — we'd rather just wait and see."

"All right. You bring her in for a checkup in a month, and then we'll know what's happening."

One month later, Inga was sprawled on the exam table. She was a magnificent, deep-bodied animal. I carefully felt her abdomen, and performed a rectal examination, but could feel no developing embryos or even an enlarged uterus.

"Well, it looks to me like she's not pregnant. It's barely possible, but at this point it seems unlikely."

Four weeks later they were back. Inga was gaining weight. As I palpated her abdomen, I could feel now what seemed to be a single fetus.

Amy and Greg looked at me with broad, knowing smiles as I announced, "Well, it looks like she's pregnant after all."

A few days later Inga gave birth to a single, huge, female puppy that weighed in at just over two pounds. She was one of the largest

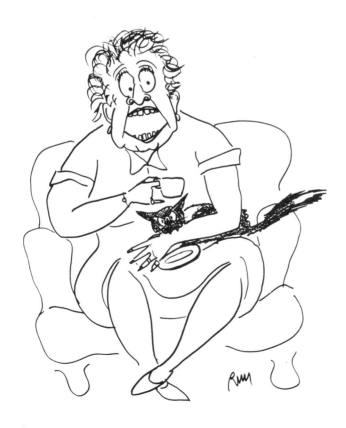

newborn puppies I have ever seen. And since her mother produced enough milk to feed a kennel, she grew almost visibly every day. She eventually grew larger than her father, Beowulf, who was himself large for the breed.

This splendid creature was a living reminder to me of my own fallibility. Not only because I saw her often, but because her owners named her Freda, in my honor!

"Hello. Dr. Frye? This is Mrs. Hudson." The woman's voice on the phone was elderly, but firm. "I wonder if you could prescribe some drug I could give my cat, to put it to sleep."

"What's the cat's trouble, Mrs. Hudson? Perhaps we can help it."

"No, no, it's beyond help. I'd prefer to put it to sleep at home, and to do it myself. A dignified, quiet death." She hesitated. "I'm quite capable of administering the drug myself. I nursed my husband for two years, until he passed away last month." There was a silence.

"How old is the cat, Mrs. Hudson?"

She seemed reluctant to reply. "I think he's three. Can you give me a prescription for something? Pills, preferably."

By this time I was fairly certain that the caller wanted the drug for herself.

"Well, Mrs. Hudson, ending a life is a serious matter. Why don't you bring the cat in here to my office, and we can talk about it."

There was a long silence, as she considered this. "All right," she said at last.

Later that afternoon, a stately woman in her seventies was ushered into my private office. She carried a wicker hamper.

"I'm Dr. Frye," I said, shaking hands. "Please sit down. Will you join me in a cup of tea?"

"Yes, thank you." she said in her strong, pleasant voice. She opened the hamper, removing a young, golden cat.

I handed her a cup of tea and reached for the animal. "So this is your cat. What do you call him?"

"We call him Toby. My husband's idea. He was very fond of him. It was his cat, actually."

"I see. And your husband just died recently, you said?"

"Yes. Last month. I — that is Toby — Toby's life is quite empty without him."

I had been giving the cat a brief examination. "He seems very healthy. Good for many years more. What he needs is a new interest. And you, too, perhaps."

"Me?" she said in her well-articulated voice. "I'm beyond the age of developing new interests. There's only one thing that life still holds for me, and that's my death. A simple, dignified death. That's all I ask."

"Well, it seems to me that you still have a lot to offer," I said. "And now that you no longer have to nurse your husband, you have the time to do it."

She took a sip of tea and looked at me uncertainly, waiting. "Your voice, for instance, is very pleasant. Have you ever considered reading aloud for the sight-impaired? I believe the library needs people to make recordings."

She was sitting up straighter in her chair, listening attentively. Toby was curled contentedly on the desk between us.

"One of my clients is the head librarian at the main library. Why don't I give her a call right now, and find out about the program?"

Mrs. Hudson nodded almost eagerly, and I dialed the number. The two women talked on the phone, and made an appointment to meet. I made a second call, to the Braille Society in Oakland, and their representative also made a date with Mrs. Hudson.

As she left, Mrs. Hudson shook my hand. "Thank you, Dr. Frye," she said, looking into my eyes. "Your advice to me and Toby is good. We will get busy again."

In the years following that cup of tea, Mrs. Hudson gave hours of her time and talent, reading books into a tape recorder so that those less fortunate than she could enjoy literature. Toby, too, lived a full, happy life.

Animals, like children, have the capacity to ingest almost anything small enough to swallow; nothing seems too vile or loathesome. Over the years we acquired an impressive collection of foreign objects retrieved from the alimentary tracts of a variety of beasts.

One afternoon a distraught couple brought in their Dachshund, which was frothing at the mouth.

"Oh, Doctor, is it rabies?" said the woman. "Just look at that foam! But he was fine just an hour ago when I got home from the grocery store."

The little dog was, indeed, frothing copiously at the mouth. The foam, however, was bright pink, and smelled strongly of soap.

"It's certainly not rabies," I said soothingly. "It looks more like some kind of soap. Is there anything he could've gotten into?"

The distracted pair could think of nothing.

"Why don't you leave Fritz here with me, and go home and make a search?"

They hurried away, and twenty minutes later the wife was on the phone.

"Dr. Frye, we're so-o-o embarrassed! We just found a chewed-up box of Brillo pads under our bed. Several pads are missing."

By this time, the soap-impregnated scouring pads had expanded in the Doxie's stomach, and had to be removed surgically.

Fritz made an uneventful recovery, and thereafter stuck to a more conventional diet!

A young woman brought in her pet boa constrictor, which had a slight bulge about midway along its length.

"It's a washcloth," she said, "I'm quite sure of it."

I could not imagine how a boa, which feeds on rats and mice, could have come to ingest a washcloth. (Or how he had had access to one, for that matter.) Perhaps his long, recurved teeth had become entangled in the fabric, and the easiest solution had been to keep swallowing.

Plain x-rays would not reveal a washcloth, since cloth is radiolucent, so my partner, Jean-Paul, administered barium directly into the stomach, via a catheter passed down the esophagus. The radiographs made after this procedure clearly showed the washcloth.

"Well," he said to the young lady, "we can operate to remove it, or we can just wait and watch. Boaz will probably either regurgitate it or eliminate it before long."

She agreed to this more conservative approach. Two weeks passed, and nothing happened. The boa was in apparent good health, but ate nothing. The bulge remained midway along the creature's length.

Four weeks passed, without any change. The snake still ate nothing, but seemed fine.

This situation continued for *ten* weeks, after which time the snake vomited a much-softened washcloth.

"That washcloth never looked so clean before!" our client laughed, as she phoned us with the good news.

After a fast of two and a half months, the snake was none the worse for wear, and neither, apparently, was the washcloth!

A young mother brought in a Pit Bull Terrier. He seemed in good health, but had been vomiting for several days.

"He has a tremendous appetite," she said, "but then he vomits it all up again."

Jean-Paul palpated the dog's abdomen, but found no suspicious masses or signs of pain. We took radiographs of the head, neck, and abdomen, but these revealed no abnormalities.

My partner and I stood looking at the dog, puzzled. The Terrier swung his head around to return our gaze, and we watched the movement. It was subtle, but the creature seemed to have some difficulty in bending his neck. As we studied him more carefully, it seemed that his head and neck were held in a slightly extended position.

"I think it's time to take a look down his throat with a gastroscope," said Jean-Paul.

We induced general anesthesia, and the tube-like gastroscope was passed down the animal's throat.

"There's something there, all right," said Jean-Paul. "Take a look."

It looked like a long dowel, just past the creature's pharynx and descending down the esophagus. At the bottom was a wooden ball. It was a xylophone mallet!

When it was removed, it measured fourteen inches. The thin reed handle had softened to the point where the dog could bend his neck almost normally. The ball on the end had acted like a check valve where the esophagus opens into the stomach.

The dog made an immediate recovery, and we returned him, and the xylophone mallet, to the happy owners.

Then there was the Boxer dog who consumed an entire package of dried barley-mushroom soup, washed it down with a hearty drink from her water bowl, and proceeded to swell up to enormous proportions. The warm moist environment of her stomach served as an efficient fermentation vat for the rapidly expanding barley. The result was a huge volume of gas, trapped in the barley mash.

Similar results are seen when dogs gain access to dry dog food, or when farm animals overeat on grain. As the gas-filled stomach expands, it puts pressure on the diaphragm, making breathing difficult. Often the stomach, spleen, esophagus and duodenum may roll or twist, cutting off blood circulation and inflow or outflow of gastric contents. It is not rare for an animal in this condition to die before it can be treated effectively.

Fortunately, the Boxer's owners were prompt in seeking emergency care. I anesthetized the dog and performed "enterogastric lavage," a procedure of flushing out the stomach and intestines similar to that performed in strychnine or snail bait poisoning. In this instance, the eight-ounce package of dried soup had swelled to several pounds of gelatinous barley mash and trapped gas.

Other items found in some of our patients were a contact lens case with the owner's lenses still inside, a matron's only set of car keys, and a valuable meerschaum pipe that did not survive its trip through the animal's alimentary system.

Some of the hardware that showed up on abdominal x-rays included coins, buttons, bobby pins, fishing hooks with swivels and sinkers attached, razor blades, nails, screws, nuts, pins, cuff links, tie tacks, rings, and wristwatches.

More of a challenge to locate or identify were various software items: baby bottle nipples and pacifiers, balloons, panty hose, a garter belt, contraceptive diaphragms and condoms, and a bikini swimsuit bra. The list is limited only by the items left unattended, and the capacity for animals to ingest the inedible!

Dogs and cats were not the only culprits. One day my client Mr. Rabinowitz brought in his large male iguana, Irving.

"I'd like you to x-ray him, Doc."

"What seems to be the trouble?"

"Well, I'm restoring this '49 Buick, and last night I was working on the carburetor on the kitchen table. The phone rings, and I go answer it. When I come back, Irving here is on the table. I get putting that thing back together, and damned if I'm not missing one screw. I *know* it was there, and I've searched high and low. So I'm thinking — maybe this guy's got it. You know — swallowed it!"

Sure enough, a radiograph showed a bevel-headed machine screw in the lizard's stomach. It was a wonderful film — even the slot in the head of the screw and the threads along the shaft were discernible.

"That's it, all right," said Mr. Rabinowitz, somewhat nonplussed. "What do we do now?"

"I think if you wait a few days, he'll deliver it," I said heartily.

He stared at the film. "I guess I'll have to work around the carburetor for now," he said stoically. "Do you remember those '49 Buicks? What great cars!"

Irving duly delivered the screw, none the worse for wear.

Another memorable offender was a female alligator from the Steinhart Aquarium. At the Aquarium's indoor alligator swamp, vis-

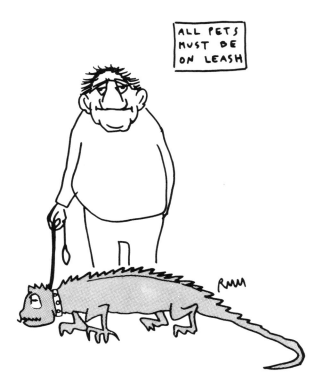

itors tossed coins into the water in hopes that their wishes would come true. The alligators watched this procedure with apparent indifference, if not outright skepticism, as they dozed on the banks.

The keepers routinely collected the coins each week, and the amounts were fairly substantial. At some point, however, they noticed that the weekly "take" was diminishing. Were people making fewer wishes? (That could only mean that Utopia was at hand!) Or was it the economy? (But no — the harder the times, the more wishes people make!)

About that time, the large female alligator seemed unwell. Her appetite had gradually declined to nothing. I was called in, and we took the creature back to the hospital in the Aquarium's van. (When we unloaded her on the stretcher, it created a small sidewalk "event," even in Berkeley, where it takes a lot to get people to stop and stare!)

Radiographs revealed a metallic lump in the alligator's abdomen. We opened her up, and found a veritable hoard of coins, and two political campaign buttons. When the coins were rinsed and counted, they amounted to several dollars. At 100 pennies to the dollar, that made for quite a load in the poor creature's stomach.

As I gazed at that heap of coins, I could not help wondering, if you make a wish and toss a coin, and that coin is eaten by an alligator, what are the implications for your wish? Being "chosen," is it more likely to come true? Or, having met with foul play, is it less likely to come true?

In the latter case, my surgical operation takes on heroic proportions. Not only did I relieve the alligator of her indigestible burden, but I also released all those hopeful wishes back into circulation!

9 | "Doctor, Could You Use Some Eggs?"

"Hello, Miss Frumkiss? This is Dr. Frye. I wanted to reassure you that Buttercup came through the surgery just fine. Incidentally, when we removed her ovaries and uterus, we discovered she was in the early stages of pregnancy. So you brought her in just in time." I always liked to make these reassuring phone calls after surgery.

There was a silence on the other end of the line, followed by a sharp intake of breath.

"What? That's impossible! Buttercup never went outdoors, and she didn't even *like* other cats!" the elderly woman fairly screamed.

"Well, perhaps Buttercup entertained a visiting tomcat," I unabashedly suggested.

Now I'd done it! The suggestion that her virgin kitten had had anything to do with some oversexed, feline Casanova only inflamed the woman more.

"You nasty man, how can you say such a thing about Buttercup? I don't ever want to speak to you again! Furthermore, you needn't send me a bill, because I have no intention of paying someone like you. And if you *do* dare to pursue this matter, I shall make a formal complaint to your local, state and national veterinary associations!"

When she paused for breath, I replied, "Madam, you are certainly entitled to your opinions. I have performed the surgery you requested, and was merely informing you of a fact in which you might be interested. Moreover, I did not charge an additional surgical fee, even though the operation took more time because of Buttercup's being in 'the family way.'"

133

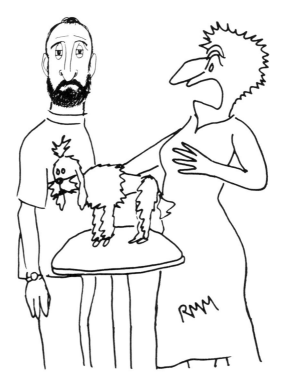

"She can't be pregnant! I'm not married!"

At that point she hung up.

A few days later we sent her a statement for a routine spay of a (slightly) pregnant cat. In four days we received a check for the full amount, but across its face was written "PAID IN PROTEST!"

I turned the check over and endorsed it "Pay to the order of the Florence Crittendon Home for Unwed Mothers," and mailed it to the Salvation Army.

Beverly had been a client of the Berkeley Dog & Cat Hospital long before I joined the staff. "Spokey," her tiny Papillon dog, was almost a fixture in the reception room. He was the center of Beverly's life, a life which had become narrower since she had lost her eyesight to severe diabetes. Before that she had been a professional photographer, and keenly interested in natural history and art. Now, Beverly got around with the help of an aluminum cane.

When Spokey first came under my care, he was ten years old, and already in cardiac decompensation and early congestive heart failure. I placed him on a low-sodium diet and medication, and his condition improved. He could once more go for short walks with his mistress.

Beverly became my particular client, and over the years we developed a very special relationship. Often, when her mother was not available to drive her to our hospital, I would make a house call after work, at her apartment in Oakland. She would talk to me as I examined Spokey, telling me how much the little brown and white dog meant to her.

"He's all I have, Dr. Frye," she said, as I moved the stethoscope over the animal's chest. "If I didn't have him, I'd have no reason to get up in the morning. Sometimes I feel that way anyway. I lie there and say, 'What's the point? Why go through the motions? Why not just end it right now? — Get it over with.'"

The first time she hinted at suicide to me, I phoned her mother, who put me in touch with the psychiatrist who saw her regularly. He, too, was concerned over her oft-expressed feelings about suicide, and her almost pathological attachment to the little dog.

Spokey's condition declined predictably over the years. When he was fourteen, I began to hint to Beverly about getting a younger companion for Spokey.

"It would be a great comfort to Spokey to have one of his own kind around. And who knows? It might give him a new lease on life."

It was Beverly who needed a new lease on life. Her depression deepened as Spokey became truly ill. One afternoon she called me.

"Dr. Frye, Spokey hasn't gotten any better. There's nothing I can do for him. He's never going to get better, and neither am I. I'm going to end my life right now."

"Beverly! Spokey needs you now as never before! You wouldn't abandon him in his hour of need, would you?"

She hesitated. "I guess you're right," she said listlessly. "I won't do it."

A few weeks later, Beverly called me. "Spokey's gone," she said calmly. "He just didn't wake up."

"I'm so sorry," I said. "May I drop by after work for a visit?"

"Fine. I'll be here."

I knocked on the door of her apartment with a certain misgiving. But Beverly was there, and offered me a cup of tea. She seemed unusually serene, and asked if I knew where she could get another Papillon puppy. I had already made several calls to breeders in the area that afternoon, but so far had come up with nothing.

One evening a week later, the phone rang at home. "It's for you," said Brucye, handing me the instrument.

"Dr. Frye? This is Beverly. I wanted to say goodbye. I've taken all my sleeping pills. It's the best way — I told you I couldn't live without Spokey."

I signalled frantically to Brucye, and scribbled a note for her to call the Oakland Fire Department on our other telephone line. I forced myself to talk calmly to Beverly.

"Beverly, I wish you hadn't done that. There's a lot of people who care about you. Are you listening to me?"

"Yes, I hear you."

"I wish you'd change your mind. It's not too late. Are you still listening?" There was a silence, followed by a clattering, as though the phone had been dropped.

"Beverly? Beverly?" There was no reply.

The police and rescue squad arrived soon afterward, broke into Beverly's apartment, and took her to a nearby hospital. She was revived, and confined overnight.

The next morning, Beverly was on the phone to me.

"You interfered! I should be free to do what I want in the privacy of my home! I didn't want all those people barging in!"

I tried to soothe her, and to interest her again in a new dog.

A week later, I had a call from Beverly's mother. "I have some bad news, Dr. Frye. Beverly took her own life last night. I thought you should know."

This time, she had called no one.

Miss Flora Coates was a cat lover. She had an undetermined number of the species, and one or another of these was frequently a patient of ours.

Miss Flora would arrive at our hospital aboard her small Honda motorbike. The cat traveled in a cardboard carton strapped on the back. Miss Flora did not wear a motorcycle helmet, but always had a scarf and heavy trench coat buttoned well below her knees, to hold her skirts in place. Straddling the motorbike was a bit cumbersome, but Miss Flora always coped.

One of the first cats of Miss Flora's that I treated had an incurable disease, and eventually died in the hospital. I called to break the inevitable news, and to ask if she'd like us to dispose of the body.

"Yes, but not yet," said Miss Flora. "I'll be bringing her home for awhile first. I'll be down in about an hour."

"All right," I said, taken aback. "We'll talk about it then."

Miss Flora stood in my office, her greying hair in disorder, her trench coat buttoned primly full length. Under her arm was the familiar cardboard box.

"Now then," I said, "tell me again what you want to do with the body. The Health Department recommends cremation, and as soon as possible. We send deceased animals to the Berkeley Animal Shelter for cremation."

"Fine. That's what I'd like. I'll have her back in three days."

I could not contain my curiosity. "In three days? What are you going to do in the meantime?"

"I will just leave her undisturbed, under my bed. After three days, her astral body will depart. Then the empty body shall be disposed of."

"I see," I said, a great overstatement.

"So tell me, Dr. Frye, when *exactly* did she die?"

I sensed the importance of this question. This was no time for vagueness or approximations. "It was at 8:10 this morning, exactly," I said firmly.

"Then at 8:10 on Sunday, her astral body will depart. I will have the *husk* here at 9:00 to be sent for cremation."

"I'm sorry, but we're not open Sunday. How about first thing Monday?"

"No, that won't do." She shook her head pityingly at my slow-wittedness. "Once the astral body is gone — after exactly three days — then the body is nothing, and must be destroyed. Isn't there a doctor on call on Sunday? I will pay for an emergency call."

I knew when I was licked. "All right, Miss Coates, someone will be here at 9:00 on Sunday." How lucky I hadn't said the cat died at midnight!

"Very good," she said, and taking the box with its unfortunate contents, she departed.

This ritual was repeated several times with various of Miss Flora's felines. The body lay in state under her bed for 72 hours, and then was brought to us for disposal. One can only imagine the accretion of astral bodies sublimed onto the underside of those bedsprings!

The Hunters were a childless couple. All the love and energy that might have been poured out on children were directed towards Igor, their cross-bred Terrier. Every year on his birthday, a resplendent party was given. Mike Hunter would pass drinks to the assembled friends, and Marla Hunter would sit beside Igor, opening his presents and expressing his thanks.

"Look, Igor! A new water dish! Now say 'thank you' to George. Thanks, George, that's great."

"Igor, a ball! A ball with a bell inside. How nice of Nancy. Say 'thank you' to Nancy, Igor."

Sometimes one of our veterinarians was among the guests, and was treated with special honors.

As the years passed, Igor's leisurely lifestyle gently aged him. Eventually he developed chronic congestive heart failure, despite our efforts with medication and a low sodium diet. One day when he was in our hospital in an oxygen cage, he died.

The Hunters had been aware that Igor had not long to live. They bore the news of his death heroically, and asked that his remains be kept in our morgue until they could make funeral arrangements. We had such facilities, and were able to comply.

A few days passed, and no word was heard from the Hunters. We transferred the body to our freezer. Weeks and then months passed, and still no word.

Finally one day, about five months after Igor's demise, his owners called.

"Hello, Dr. Frye? This is Mike Hunter. About Igor — you do still have him, don't you?"

"Yes, we do. But we can't keep him forever. I hope you've made some arrangements."

"I'm sorry about the delay. The thing is, we've been trying to find a taxidermist who will fix Igor up. We wanted to keep him in the living room — sitting up on his hindlegs with a ball, or something cute, you know. You've seen that kind of thing at the natural history museum, haven't you? They look almost alive."

He paused, and sighed heavily. "The trouble is, nobody's willing to do it. We've tried everywhere. But we'll come up with something, if you can just wait a little longer."

"Mike, I think it's too late for that. He's been dead too long. Why don't you get a nice box and bury him?"

He was silent, and I held my breath. "I'll talk to Marla," he said finally, "and be back in touch. We'll think of something."

Two months later, the Hunters arrived at the hospital with a custom-made, satin-lined casket. Igor's remains were transferred to this, and closed from sight. They buried him with ceremony on a hillside where his grave could be visited by those who loved him.

We were all relieved to see Igor go to his final resting place. As to the style of his going — who can sit in judgment on the emotions and deep attachments of others?

One sunny afternoon Clarke Atwater appeared in the doorway of my office, where I was going over some records.

"I wish you'd give me a hand here, Fred," he said, glancing over his shoulder and lowering his voice.

"I've got this young woman in the exam room with two dogs, a German Shepherd and a St. Bernard. The dogs have got mange — I checked out some skin scrapings under the microscope, and it's *Sarcoptes scabei*, no doubt about it. The thing is . . ." He hesitated, and looked embarrassed.

"Well?" I said encouragingly.

"She asked me if the mites could be transmitted to humans, and when I said 'yes,' she said she's got some itchy places too. She said . . ." Clarke glanced behind him again and leaned forward. "She said she likes to wrestle with her dogs, in the *nude!*" He looked at me helplessly.

"Well, well, this could be very interesting. Medically, that is," I said. "Would you like me to join you as a consultant in pursuing this case?"

Clarke gulped visibly. "I'd appreciate it, Fred."

The client was sitting comfortably in the exam room, with her two dogs at her feet. She wore blue jeans and a peasant-style blouse. Reddish curly hair protruded from under a bandana.

"Well now," I said affably, "Dr. Atwater tells me that these two fellows have mites. Let's have a look."

"They sure do," she said. "And so do I, all over here." She lifted the blouse a few inches and displayed an expanse of reddened skin.

"This is an interesting case," I said. "Would you mind if I took photographs of the dogs' lesions, and yours?"

"My what?" she said uncertainly.

"The area of inflamed skin," I said reassuringly.

"Oh. Sure. No sweat."

"Let's go outside in the patio," I said to Clarke. "The light's better out there."

Our back patio was secluded from the street, but was overlooked by apartments. We ushered the client and her dogs through the library and out the sliding glass door.

"Okay, Clarke, if you'll just hold the St. Bernard there," I said, focusing my camera.

"See, it's real bad up here," said the young woman's voice behind me, and I saw Clarke's face blanch.

I turned to find that our client had completely shucked her blouse, and was now standing naked from the waist up in full view of all the neighboring apartments.

Recovering from my surprise, I bent my attention to our scientific endeavors. She had, in fact, the worst case of human scabies I have ever seen. Hardly a square centimeter of her skin was without tiny blisters.

"How long have you had this condition?" I asked as I focused on a particularly inflamed lesion.

"A couple of months," she said.

"Did it start about the same time as the dogs' itchiness?" I prompted.

"No, it seems like I got it first," she said, turning her face up to enjoy the sun.

"I see."

"Maybe I gave it to them?" she suggested idly.

"It could be possible," I admitted.

"Oh. I never thought of that before."

After she had put on her blouse and departed, Clarke looked at me.

"Well!" I said slapping him on the back. "And I always thought dermatology was boring!"

"But. . ." said Clarke, still stunned. He gestured to the apartments. "I wonder how many people were watching? I mean, she didn't even seem to *care*! And who does she think we are, that she goes stripping in front of us?"

"Doctors, my dear boy, doctors!" I said, straightening the collar of my white coat. "It's all the same thing. She knew she was in the hands of professionals."

"Hmph," said Clarke. "I think I'll stick with cats and dogs."

"You're wise," I said, and we both laughed.

It was a mellow Saturday evening at the home of our friends the Horikoshis. Wonderful smells emanated from the kitchen. Brucye smiled at me across the candlelight, and we all raised our sake cups. Just then the telephone rang.

"It's for you," our hostess said. "It's your answering service."

Groaning inwardly, I excused myself to the kitchen.

"Hi, Dr. Frye? There's this guy on the phone. He says it's not an emergency, but that you won't regret it if you talk to him."

This was too much for my curiosity. "Okay, I'll take it." Wrapped in the delicious aroma emanating from the hibachi, I waited.

"Evenin' doctor," said the drawling voice. "Could you use some eggs?"

I was taken off guard. "*Free* eggs," the voice continued.

"What kind of eggs?" I said, making a recovery. "And why are you calling me about it *now*?"

"Hell, doc, they're chicken eggs! I just thought you could use 'em. They won't keep."

"How many eggs do you have?" I parried.

"Quite a few."

"Well look," I said, inhaling the scent of teriyaki, "I'll call the hospital and have the night watchman let you bring them into our walk-in refrigerator. I'm sure we'd all appreciate having them, and what we can't eat we'll feed to the dogs and cats. Thanks for thinking of us."

"Doc, you don't understand," he said. "You've gotta have something to put them in — they're not in their shells. And they've been kinda *used*, so they can't be eaten by people, but the animals should love 'em. There are ninety dozen of them."

At this point my curiosity overcame my gourmandise. I decided I could slip away for a few minutes and be back shortly, no doubt with a tale to tell.

"Okay," I said to the caller, "I'm only a few blocks from the hospital. I'll meet you there."

Brucye and Elliot and Joan Horikoshi were as intrigued as I when I recounted this conversation, and they exused me with good grace.

As I drove over there, I tried to guess what anyone would be doing with the contents of ninety dozen hens' eggs. I had not yet grasped that this was 1080 eggs! I innocently assumed that a few stainless steel surgery pails and pans would do the job.

My benefactor was waiting in the parking lot, with the sliding door of his van open. Inside was a 30-gallon garbage can.

"Hi, doc. Here it is! It's too heavy to carry — we'll have to ladle it out into your containers."

The garbage can was brimming with scrambled, golden fluid.

I was staggered, but rallied quickly. Enlisting Johnny's aid, I rounded up every spare pail, pan, jar or vessel I could find, and lined them up on the pavement around the van.

The fellow and I began ladling the stuff into this flotilla, and carrying it into our morgue refrigerator. Johnny accepted this influx without question. After a few trips, though, my curiosity could be contained no longer.

"What in blazes were you doing with all these eggs?" I asked as a basinful slopped onto my sleeve.

"Well doc, it's like, we were shooting a flick in the woods. Under these pine trees. We had to have this bathtub full of beaten eggs. *"You know,"* he leered at me, "the *primeval* scene!"

"You mean a skin flick?"

"You got it!" He smiled knowingly.

I digested this in silence as we made another trip to the morgue.

"But the eggs — how did you *do* it?" I asked as he ladled the stuff into the coffee pot I was holding.

"Well, man, it took *time*," he said with a touch of pride. "We just sat there and cracked and emptied, cracked and emptied. When we got tired, we'd take a little rest, smoke a joint, and then get back to it. When we were all done, we stirred it up with a board."

As the tale unfolded, it appeared that into this slimy mess was lowered the heroine of the cinematic epic! (What exactly ensued was not divulged, nor did I feel I should ask. Later, I watched the local theatre listings for this sylvan idyll, but to no avail.)

We were nearing the bottom of the barrrel. "Are you sure you don't want to keep some for yourself?" I asked. "You don't have a dog or a cat?"

"Naw," he said. "Besides, I don't ever want to see an egg again."

A few moments later, he shook my hand and drove off into the night. Johnny and I stowed the last bit of provender and washed our hands.

"Well now, I don't quite ken what yon fella was doin' with all th'eggs," said Johnny.

"Up to no good," I said with a wink. "You wouldn't believe what some people do for entertainment."

"Ah, is that how it is?" said Johnny. "Well now, imagine that. Well, the wee beasties will enjoy it, surrrely."

Back at the dinner party, the smell of grilled chicken teriyaki still lingered on the air. Elliot and Joan and Brucye greeted me with eager questions and incredulity. As I sat over my reheated dinner, the four of us discussed ways of dealing with the eggs. Freeze them? Cook them? Dump them? (But where?)

While this problem still lay unsolved, we passed on to more entertaining speculations, about the exact scenario there beneath the whispering pines.

"So what did they *do* in this bathtub full of eggs?" giggled Brucye.

"Naughty things, I'm sure," I said.

"Oh. How awful for the heroine! And she probably had to drive all the way back to town before she could get a real bath. Poor girl!"

"Think of her clothes!" said Joan, taking up this theme. "You know, there is a glue made from raw egg. Her clothes were probably glued on hard by the time she got home."

"She could soak them off in a warm tub," said Brucye reassuringly. "I'm sure it would work."

Elliot and I looked at each other, and we all laughed.

On Monday morning, I explained our windfall to the rest of the staff. After a few moments of open-mouthed disbelief, they rose to the occasion nobly.

We rejected the idea of freezing the eggs after trying it on a small sample. The thawed eggs separated into a disgusting, runny mess. The only alternative was to cook them.

Brucye took command, borrowed as many electric skillets as she could, and mobilized the staff in shifts. Not even licensed veterinarians were exempt.

Soon the smell of cooking eggs permeated the entire hospital. Naturally our clients were curious about the smell, and we gave out a slightly abridged version of the tale.

Everyone took thirty-minute turns at the frying pans, after which it was necessary to run outside and gulp in fresh air. This routine went on for several days, as was reflected in our subsequent electric bill. The cooled batches of eggs were packed in plastic bags and frozen.

Long after the cooking process was finally completed, a sulfurous residuum lingered in the vicinity of the kitchen and lounge. The dogs and cats who were fed the eggs as part of their daily fare seemed to enjoy their share of the former bubble bath. As for the rest of us, it was a long time before any of us could contemplate eating an egg!

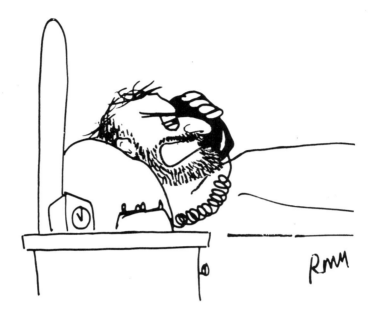

"Hello? ....Am I at the office? ....Certainly I am. I sleep on the operating table!"

One night I was sleeping peacefully, when the telephone shrilled its way into my slumbers.

"Doc, I gotta know the anshwer to thish queshtion," said the slurred voice in my ear. "It'sh been buggin' me for years. Me and the boys here have a bet on it, and you gotta shettle it for ush." There was a pause, and I could hear encouraging shouts in the background.

"The queshtion is thish: is a tiger *black* with *orange* stripesh, or" — I could almost hear him sorting out his befuddled wits — "*orange* with *black* stripesh?"

"Well," I said grimly, "I will have to do a bit of research on this. Please give me your name, address, and phone number, and I'll get back to you as soon as I can."

He was obviously too drunk to see what was coming, for he dutifully gave me all the information. I set my alarm for 5:30 and went back to sleep.

At 5:30, I dialed the number. It rang for a long time, and finally a man's groggy voice answered.

"Hello, Mr. Welch? This is Dr. Frye, returning your call. You wanted to know about the tiger's stripes?" My voice was brisk and cheerful.

"Huh? Hmm? Uh--yeah?" These sounds were music to my ears.

"Well, it has taken me awhile to research this, but I have the answer for you."

"Mmm . . . Umm . . . Yeah?" I detected a rising level of alertness in these noises. "Yeah? So which way is it, doc?"

"In my opinion, tigers are decorated with *alternating* stripes of black and orange."

"Alternating?"

"That's right."

There was a long pause. "That's a good answer," he said finally. "Nobody will ever get that one right. Thanks, doc."

"My office will be sending you a bill for professional services," I said, "including the usual after-hours emergency fee."

"Okay, doc." And he hung up.

A few days later his check for the full amount arrived, along with a handwritten note which read:

Dear Dr. Frye:

> *It was worth 30 bucks for me to get the answer to that tiger question. It's been bugging me for years. Glad you've got a good sense of humor.*

> *Yours,*
> *Ray Welch*

I endorsed the check over to CARE, with a satisfied feeling that justice had been done. I'm sure that my nocturnal caller used that answer to win many, many beer bets.

It was the end of a long day, and on my exam table was an emergency case. It was a gopher tortoise with a badly damaged shell, bound up with masking tape.

"Oh, I feel so terrible," said the young woman standing beside me. "It's all my fault. I was practicing a dance routine in my apartment, and I tripped over him. I fell right on top of him, and my skin got pinched between the broken pieces of his shell. I had to have some stitches." She raised her thigh into view, and displayed a bandaged area. "See?"

I saw not only this, but the rest of her charms which were amply displayed by her costume: short pink "hot pants," and a filmy see-through blouse.

"Well now," I said, tearing my eyes away from this visual feast, and returning them to the hapless tortoise. "Let's see what we can do for this fellow."

There were several shell fractures, and blood was dripping from them. I cleansed these with antiseptic solution.

"I think I can patch him back together with fiberglass and epoxy resin," I reassured the young woman.

"Can you? That would be super! I'm crazy about him. His name is Horace."

"Well, you leave Horace with me, and call in tomorrow to see how he's doing."

"Thanks, Dr. Frye. I've got to get going. I've got to call the club and tell them I won't be performing tonight."

"You're a dancer?" I said politely.

She nodded. "Go-go dancing. Over at the Casbah Club. You ever been there?"

"No. I'm afraid I've never seen go-go dancing," I admitted regretfully.

"No kidding! Well, you'll have to drop by the club sometime. You don't know what you're missing!"

I repaired the tortoise successfully, and the next morning he was awake and eating strawberries.

The young woman was very grateful when she was reunited with her pet.

"I'll tell you what," she said eagerly. "In about two weeks, I should be back dancing again, and I'd like you and your wife to be my guests at the club. You said you'd never seen go-go-dancing. So here's your chance!"

On a subsequent Saturday night, Brucye and I were ushered to a select table adjoining the dance floor, at the Casbah Club.

"Nothing but the best," said Brucye, laughing, after a steward had seated us and departed. "People will think you're some Hollywood agent, not the star's veterinarian!"

"What's wrong with being her veterinarian?" I countered. "A respectable profession."

"But of course!" said Brucye. "You're probably the most respectable person here tonight."

I glanced around at the darkened tables. "Except for you, of course," I said gallantly.

"Well, maybe so," Brucye conceded, and we both laughed.

Soon the entertainment began. My client and two other scantily clad damsels appeared and began the prancing movements of go-go dancing.

"There she is," I whispered to Brucye. "The one with dark hair."

"Ah. I see," said Brucye, watching intently.

The rhythmic beat of the music accelerated, and the trio pranced faster and faster. My client threw dazzling smiles in our direction, and spent several steamy minutes gyrating a few feet from our table.

"I thought you said she'd had stitches in her thigh," said Brucye, as the dancer moved away. "I didn't see anything."

"She seems to have made a good recovery," I agreed, "just like her tortoise. She must have a good doctor."

"As well as a good veterinarian," said Brucye, laughing.

"I'm glad you think so!" I sat back and surveyed the scene. "You know, veterinary medicine has some amazing fringe benefits. Like right now. It's gotten us the best table in the house here at the Casbah Club."

"And don't forget the eighty pounds of whale meat," said Brucye. "Another unexpected windfall!"

"You're right," I said seriously. "You never know what's coming next." I leaned back in my chair and smiled at my wife. "It's not a bad life, being a veterinarian."

"Or being married to a veterinarian," she responded. We smiled at each other.

"No," I repeated, "It's not a bad life at all."

Epilogue I

I sold my practice and the Berkeley Dog & Cat Hospital in 1976, after buying my partner's share three years before. Two years after the expedition to the Indus, I had been hospitalized for a serious parasite infestation I'd acquired there. After having my appendix, spleen and part of my liver and diaphragm removed, I resumed practice. However, I was hospitalized four more times in the next four years for problems related to this.

The final decision to sell the practice was a difficult one to make. The practice had occupied most of my energies and time for the past ten years; it had been the main source of my family's income; and was kind to my ego. Our clients were grand, and many had become close personal friends. (When some of them learned of my hospitalization and impending major surgery, they spontaneously organized a blood drive for me.) The staff at the hospital had been together for many years, and had been wonderfully supportive of the practice and of me. Most of them stayed on with the new owners, and so I left the Berkeley Dog & Cat Hospital knowing that my patients and clients would continue to be well-served by dedicated people.

That summer, Brucye and I and our teenaged children spent three months aboard our houseboat in the Sacramento-San Joaquin River delta system. I worked on a second veterinary medical textbook (*Biomedical and Surgical Aspects of Captive Reptile Husbandry*) and relaxed and unwound from my former lifestyle of eighty-hour work weeks.

The following year we moved back to Davis, and I re-entered the university as a graduate student in comparative pathology. We spent the next summer aboard the houseboat again, while I studied for the comprehensive examination. I earned my Master's degree that August.

149

Since then, I have worked as a consultant in veterinary medicine and surgery, and in institutional comparative medicine and histopathology. I have also served as a clinical professor of medicine at the Veterinary School at Davis, and have done work in photomicroscopy and photomacroscopy. I have written chapters for textbooks, and many scientific articles.

As I gain perspective on my years in practice, I realize more and more that technical brilliance alone can not make a successful practice; the ability to enter into the feelings of clients is just as important, if not more so. For many a lonely pet owner, the veterinarian sometimes serves as advisor, confidant, and even confessor, on a range of subjects that may have little to do with the animal being treated.

My time spent working with animals and people has been very gratifying. Years ago, when I was still aspiring to be a veterinarian, I came across some verses by Walt Whitman that well express the kind of contentment that can come from working closely with creatures:

I think I could turn and live with animals, they are
*   so placid and self-contain'd,*
I stand and look at them long and long.
They do not sweat and whine about their condition,
They do not lie awake in the dark and weep for
*   their sins,*
They do not make me sick discussing their duty
*   to God,*
Not one is dissatisfied, not one is demented with
*   the mania of owning things,*
Not one kneels to another, nor to his kind that
*   lived thousands of years ago,*
Not one is respectable or unhappy over the whole
*   earth.*

"Song of Myself," in
Leaves of Grass

Epilogue II

In the intervening 10 years since the first edition of this book was written and published and this new edition was published, several important changes have occurred in clinical veterinary medicine in North America and Europe: There has been a substantial increase in the number of women who have chosen to study and practice veterinary medicine; and the type of animals, particularly in urban areas, has significantly changed from one where the vast majority were dogs and cats to the situation today where almost any creature that walks, crawls, flies or swims is treated by modern family-practice oriented veterinarians. In my opinion, the addition of women to veterinary medicine has greatly enhanced our profession's effectiveness and image with the public. As the profession has matured, many specialties and subspecialties became viable alternatives to more conventional small-companion animal and large farm-type animal practices. There are now veterinarians whose practices are strictly limited to ornamental fish, reptiles and amphibians, caged birds, miniature pigs, or "pocket pets" such as hamsters, gerbils, guinea pigs, rabbits, chinchillas, ferrets, hedgehogs, sugar gliders, etc. Even the number of invertebrates such as tarantulas, scorpions, praying mantids, colorful aquarium and terrestrial hermit crabs, and snails kept as "pets" has increased substantially during the last decade.

When I began practicing clinical veterinary medicine in January 1966, many of my colleagues thought I was foolish to spend so much time on reptiles, amphibians, small rodents, zoo cats, primates, spiders, snails, etc. I was warned by more than one of my colleagues that my forays into providing medical and surgical care for exotic "pet" animals would result in my losing ever-increasing income because (1) a practice limited to dogs and cats would be much more lucrative and (2) the "learning curve" (a term new to our lexicon) was very steep because there was so little published information

151

regarding and so few knowledgeable colleagues engaged in treating small non-domestic animals. During that time some of the few experienced clinicians who were invited to give seminars often kept their "secrets" to themselves in the mistaken belief that to let others know about their practice methods would only create competitors! Many of us who began accepting "exotic" animals as patients three decades ago did so with little or no formal training and, as a consequence, did not charge for our services until we were confident that we possessed sufficient expertise to justify our fees. Several years after I had begun treating exotic animals, I still was not charging a fee; I asked my clients to make a donation to CARE in lieu of paying me because when I was a medical officer with the Smithsonian Institution's expedition to (West) Pakistan in 1968, I witnessed CARE actually providing the services for which they claimed credit, and I was impressed with their effectiveness. In the meantime, I (and my partner, Dr. Jean-Paul E. Cucuel) subsidized many of the fees that were necessary in order to diagnose and treat some exotic animal patients (laboratory fees charged to an animal hospital are the same whether or not the patient is a dog, cat, horse, parrot, or turtle—the extrinsic monetary value of the patient has no bearing on the fees, nor should it, because the expenses incurred are equal). Finally, after I believed that I possessed sufficient proficiency, I commenced charging professional fees.

Surprisingly, the increased curiosity regarding the biology, captive behavior, husbandry, nutrition, and medical and surgical management of so-called "exotic" or non-traditional creatures has been fulfilled primarily not by the established schools and colleges of veterinary medicine but, rather, by local, state, and national veterinary medical associations and professional special interest groups who sponsor erudite lectures and seminars, and by well-informed and experienced veterinarians who are willing and able to teach their colleagues the art of treating these unusual patients. There is now a parallel situation in the veterinary profession to what is found within the medical profession: Veterinary clinicians interested in enhancing their proficiency in "expert" areas of practice can take advantage of formal educational training offered by specialty boards and colleges which ensure a high degree of quality.

There is a modicum of truth in the observation that veterinarians may be expected to serve as unpaid—or very poorly recompensed— psychotherapists for some of their clients. An understanding sympathetic ear and the trappings of medicine (a stethoscope, the appellation "Dr.," being a member of the healing arts, etc.) make for a natural transference. However, rarely are veterinarians adequately prepared for assuming the mantle that such a role demands. Calling upon logic usually is not a successful defense against these onslaughts. I am reminded of Dr. Daniel E. Koshland's observation* that, "The gene for unbridled dedication to a lost cause will always overwhelm the pure logic gene."

Some animals are in such poor condition that even the most heroic measures cannot save their lives. I have observed persons who, when given the alternative selection of a healthy puppy or kitten, or a pot-bellied, obviously wormy, lethargic runt of the litter, will unhesitatingly choose the latter. Similarly, some amateur herpetologists will purposely select underfed, deformed, listless reptiles from a group of much more healthy individuals on display at a pet store. Frequently, this is done because the well-meaning person believes that no one else would take in such a waif and it would surely die. This behavior is highly laudable, but it often leads to repeated frustration because by the time that many reptiles reach the retail end of the prolonged exotic animal distribution chain, they have been so stressed by shipment, exposure to parasites and infectious diseases, poor nutrition, and dehydration that it would take a miracle to return them to health. In the process, much time and money is spent on what may result in a losing cause and disappointment. "Do whatever it takes Doc—and don't spare the expense" is the plea of the owner. Whether the outcome is positive or negative, when the time comes to collect for even the materials alone, the client's tune may change to one of recrimination. (Some clients expect veterinarians to be content with only the intellectual challenges and not be overly concerned with paying for the mortgages, salaries, taxes, license fees, groceries, etc. These expectations may be justified because the challenges *are* intensely interesting and, besides, if we were *really* interested in accumulating wealth, we have chosen the wrong profession to accomplish that goal.)

One feature of exotic animal practice that definitely has not changed is the often bizarre behavior exhibited by many people who choose to keep caged and uncaged reptiles and other so-called "lower" animals. Whether these behavioral patterns are already well ingrained *before* exotic animal owners obtain their pets or whether by virtue of keeping reptiles or other wild animals this odd behavior is induced is conjectural. However, a pattern has emerged.

The favorite reptilian pet of the 1990's is the common green iguana. This vigorous, flamboyant, relatively intelligent (for a reptile) lizard can, with appropriate nutrition and husbandry, live for more than 20 years. In many homes, pet iguanas dine with their owners, bathe with their owners, and sleep with their owners. Iguanas living

*Science, 265:1639, 1994.

in southern California, Texas, and Florida may be adorned with shiny gold chains; iguanas living in more northern climes may be outfitted with cozy colorful sweaters and hats. The iguana's birthday may be a festive occasion celebrated with (of course) a birthday cake (optimally made from vegetables and fruit) replete with decorations and the correct number of candles!

Although perceived by the general public as being "weird," the majority of exotic animal owners are devoted to providing the best care possible for their unusual pets. On one occasion when Brucye and I were in New York visiting our daughter, son-in-law, and grandson, we were about to depart from our hotel room when there was a knock at the door. Upon answering the summons, I found a young man holding a small, blind diamondback terrapin. Somehow, he knew that I was in New York and was anxious to show me his special pet. With enthusiasm and pride, he explained how he had been hand-feeding little periwinkle snails that he had gathered in Long Island Sound for the terrapin for several months. I am entirely confident that without his owner's dedication, the little terrapin whose eyes had never formed would have starved to death. Today, over 7 years later, that terrapin is nearly fully grown and continues to take tender morsels from the fingers of his sensitive and committed owner.

During over 30 years of research and practice, I have gained a deep appreciation for the human:animal bond that develops between a pet owner and his or her cherished animal companion. I believe that these close bonds are strengthened through mutually beneficial interrelationships between a human and a non-judgmental animal. When I was in full-time companion animal practice, the most difficult problem I ever confronted was when I had to gently inform an elderly person that his or her much-loved—and needed—dog or cat had a terminal condition. It was a wrenching experience for my trusting clients and for me. Obviously, we made every effort to keep these animals alive and pain-free (as humanly and as humanely possible). To give my readers an example of such a close human:animal bond, I am reproducing a verbatim copy of a letter that I received very shortly after the first edition of this book was published. It was written in a shaky handwriting and it clearly illustrates the deep love and devotion this elderly lady had for her Sheltie dog.

"Dear Dr. Frye,

Thanks for sending a letter informing me where I could get your book. I'm going to include it when I give my daughter her birthday gifts.

May I tell you about our little fellow. I'm in a wheelchair, so two years ago, our daughter placed a 3-month-old Sheltie puppy in my lap. He is rust-colored with a snow-white chest; thus I named him 'Rusty.' When he tried to chew on my fingers, I said 'Don't bite me!' He quickly learned to be very careful. He found a strap hanging from the cushion behind my wheelchair a fine thing to chew on—and if he pulled, he could back me and my chair up.

An Animal 'shrink' on radio station KGO said that dogs only understand 3 words. That is false.

In the mornings my husband, Frank, says 'Time to get Mama up!' and Rusty comes barking down the hall to wake me. At night, Frank says 'Time for little dogs to go potty' and he walks to the door, then he lets out a tiny 'yip' when he's done.

Mornings Rusty sits beside me to get cereal flakes which he chews instead of gulping down like most dogs. He eats the last 2 spoonsful of my cereal off a spoon. Evenings he gets a bit of meat daintly removed from his own fork. After my cereal, he and Frank go get the newspaper; then he hurries back for his little piece of my toast and jelly.

We keep stamps in a plastic box; when Rusty hears the box snap open, he can hardly wait to go to the mailbox.

At the mention of our daughter's dog's name, Rusty goes right to the front door waiting for her arrival! Of course, he knows many words, so we spell things when we don't want him to know what we are saying.

Frank and I feel that Rusty is bilingual because he understands English, speaks Dog—for the strangest noises come out of him, from a doggie bark at various levels, to all sorts of howls and moans—and every sound in between.

Dr. Frye, we sure enjoy and love our little boy. He really enjoys being told that 'he's a good boy.' If you ever write another book, you may use any of this; animals are a real delight."

                                        Thanks again,
                                        Mrs. R. G.

Mrs. R. G. said it all: Animals *are* a real delight—and so are their owners!